Praise for

THE GOOD LIFE

"Robert Waldinger and Marc Schulz lead us on an empowering quest toward our greatest need: meaningful human connection. Blending research from an ongoing eighty-year study of life satisfaction with emotional storytelling proves that ancient wisdom has been right all along—a good life is built with good relationships."

—Jay Shetty, bestselling author of *Think Like a Monk* and host of the podcast *On Purpose*

"In a crowded field of life advice, and even life advice based on scientific research, Schulz and Waldinger stand apart. Capitalizing on the most intensive study of adult development in history, they tell us what makes a good life and why."

—Angela Duckworth, bestselling author of *Grit*; Rosa Lee and Egbert Chang Professor, University of Pennsylvania; and cofounder, chief scientist, and board member of Character Lab

"Want the secret to the good life? Waldinger and Schulz give it to you in this magnificent new book. Based on the longest survey ever conducted over people's lives, *The Good Life* reveals who winds up happy, who doesn't, and why—and how you can use this information, starting today."

—Arthur C. Brooks, professor, Harvard Kennedy School and Harvard Business School, and #1 *New York Times* bestselling author

"Waldinger and Schulz are world experts on the counterintuitive things that make life meaningful. Their book will provide welcome advice for a world facing unprecedented levels of unhappiness and loneliness."

—Laurie Santos, Chandrika and Ranjan Tandon Professor of Psychology, Yale University, and host of *The Happiness Lab* podcast

"*The Good Life* tells the story of a rare and fascinating study of lives over time. This insightful, interesting, and well-informed book reveals the secret of happiness and reminds us that it was never really a secret after all."

—Daniel Gilbert, author of the *New York Times*
bestseller *Stumbling on Happiness* and host
of the PBS television series *This Emotional Life*

"Waldinger and Schulz have written an essential—perhaps *the* essential—book on human flourishing. Backed by extraordinary research and packed with actionable advice, *The Good Life* will expand your brain and enrich your heart."

—Daniel H. Pink, #1 *New York Times* bestselling author
of *The Power of Regret*, *Drive*, and *A Whole New Mind*

"I'm beyond thrilled that Waldinger and Schulz are publishing the findings of the Harvard Study. Over the years, I've discussed their research and recommended Waldinger's TED Talk around the world. I can hardly wait to recommend *The Good Life*. The book is accessible, interesting, and grounded in research—and is bound to make a difference in the lives of millions."

—Tal Ben-Shahar, bestselling author
of *Being Happy: You Don't Have to Be Perfect to Lead a Richer, Happier Life*
and *Happier: Learn the Secrets to Daily Joy and Lasting Fulfillment*

"This book is simply extraordinary. It weaves 'hard data' and enlightening case studies and interviews together seamlessly in a way that stays true to the science while humanizing it. And what an important lesson it teaches. It helps people to understand how they should live their lives and also provides a spectacular picture of what psychology can be at its best. It is data driven, of course, but data are just noise without wise interpretation."

—Barry Schwartz, coauthor of *Practical Wisdom*
and author of *Why We Work*

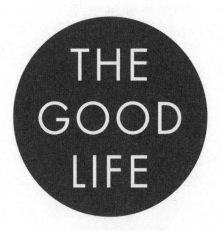

THE GOOD LIFE

Lessons from the World's Longest
Scientific Study of Happiness

ROBERT WALDINGER, MD
and MARC SCHULZ, PhD

SIMON & SCHUSTER
New York   London   Toronto   Sydney   New Delhi

Simon & Schuster
1230 Avenue of the Americas
New York, NY 10020

First Simon & Schuster hardcover edition January 2023

SIMON & SCHUSTER and colophon are registered trademarks of Simon & Schuster, Inc.

For information about special discounts for bulk purchases, please contact
Simon & Schuster Special Sales at 1-866-506-1949 or business@simonandschuster.com.

The Simon & Schuster Speakers Bureau can bring authors to your live event.
For more information or to book an event, contact the Simon & Schuster Speakers Bureau
at 1-866-248-3049 or visit our website at www.simonspeakers.com.

Interior design by Ruth Lee-Mui

Manufactured in the United States of America

5   7   9   10   8   6   4

Library of Congress Cataloging-in-Publication Data is available.

ISBN 978-1-9821-6669-4
ISBN 978-1-9821-6671-7 (ebook)

*To the families we were born into
and the families we helped create*

CONTENTS

AUTHORS' NOTE

The Harvard Study of Adult Development has followed the lives of two generations of individuals from the same families for more than eighty years. Shepherding a study like this requires tremendous trust. Part of that trust comes from a deep commitment to protecting the confidentiality of participants. We have changed names and identifying details to protect participants' confidentiality. All quotes in the book, however, are either verbatim or based on actual study interviews, audiotapes, observations, and other data.

1

WHAT MAKES A GOOD LIFE?

There isn't time, so brief is life, for bickerings, apologies, heartburn-
ings, callings to account. There is only time for loving, and but an
instant, so to speak, for that.

Mark Twain

Let's begin with a question:

If you had to make *one* life choice, right now, to set yourself on the
path to future health and happiness, what would it be?

Would you choose to put more money into savings each month? To
change careers? Would you decide to travel more? What single choice
could best ensure that when you reach your final days and look back,
you'll feel that you've lived a good life?

In a 2007 survey, millennials were asked about their most important
life goals. Seventy-six percent said that becoming rich was their number
one goal. Fifty percent said a major goal was to become famous. More
than a decade later, after millennials had spent more time as adults, similar questions were asked again in a pair of surveys. Fame was now lower
on the list, but the top goals again included things like making money,
having a successful career, and becoming debt-free.

These are common and practical goals that extend across generations and borders. In many countries, from the time they are barely old enough to speak, children are asked what they want to be when they grow up—that is, what careers they intend to pursue. When adults meet new people, one of the first questions asked is, "What do you do?" Success in life is often measured by title, salary, and recognition of achievement, even though most of us understand that these things do not necessarily make for a happy life on their own. Those who manage to check off some or even all of the desired boxes often find themselves on the other side feeling much the same as before.

Meanwhile, all day long we're bombarded with messages about what will make us happy, about what we should want in our lives, about who is doing life "right." Ads tell us that eating this brand of yogurt will make us healthy, buying that smartphone will bring new joy to our lives, and using a special face cream will keep us young forever.

Other messages are less explicit, woven into the fabric of daily living. If a friend buys a new car, we might wonder if a newer car would make our own life better. As we scroll social media feeds seeing only pictures of fantastic parties and sandy beaches, we might wonder if our own life is lacking in parties, lacking in beaches. In our casual friendships, at work, and especially on social media, we tend to show each other idealized versions of ourselves. We present our game faces, and the comparison between what we *see* of each other and how we *feel* about ourselves leaves us with the sense that we're missing out. As an old saying goes, *We are always comparing our insides to other people's outsides.*

Over time we develop the subtle but hard-to-shake feeling that our life is *here*, now, and the things we need for a good life are *over there*, or in the future. Always just out of reach.

Looking at life through this lens, it's easy to believe that the good life doesn't really exist, or else that it's only possible for others. Our own life, after all, rarely matches the picture we've created in our heads of what a good life should look like. Our own life is always too messy, too complicated to be good.

Spoiler alert: The good life *is* a complicated life. For everybody.

The good life is joyful . . . and challenging. Full of love, but also pain. And it never strictly *happens*; instead, the good life *unfolds*, through time. It is a process. It includes turmoil, calm, lightness, burdens, struggles, achievements, setbacks, leaps forward, and terrible falls. And of course, the good life always ends in death.

A cheery sales pitch, we know.

But let's not mince words. Life, even when it's good, is not easy. There is simply no way to make life perfect, and if there were, then it wouldn't be good.

Why? *Because a rich life—a good life—is forged from precisely the things that make it hard.*

This book is built on a bedrock of scientific research. At its heart is the Harvard Study of Adult Development, an extraordinary scientific endeavor that began in 1938, and against all odds is still going strong today. Bob is the fourth director of the Study, and Marc its associate director. Radical for its time, the Study set out to understand human health by investigating not what made people sick, but what made them thrive. It has recorded the experience of its participants' lives more or less as they were happening, from childhood troubles, to first loves, to final days. Like the lives of its participants, the Harvard Study's road has itself been long and winding, evolving in its methods over the decades and expanding to now include three generations and more than 1,300 of the descendants of its original 724 participants. It continues to evolve and expand today, and is the longest in-depth longitudinal study of human life ever done.

But no single study, no matter how rich, is enough to permit broad claims about human life. So while this book stands directly on the foundation of the Harvard Study, it is supported on all sides by hundreds of other scientific studies involving many thousands of people from all over the world. The book is also threaded with wisdom from the recent and ancient past—enduring ideas that mirror and enrich modern scientific understandings of the human experience. It is a book primarily about the power of relationships, and it is deeply informed, appropriately, by the long and fruitful friendship of its authors.

But the book would not exist without the human beings who took part in the Harvard Study's research—whose honesty and generosity made this unlikely study possible in the first place.

People like Rosa and Henry Keane.

"What is your greatest fear?"

Rosa read the question out loud and then looked across the kitchen table at her husband, Henry. Now in their 70s, Rosa and Henry had lived in this house and sat at this same table together on most mornings for more than fifty years. Between them sat a pot of tea, an open pack of Oreos (half eaten), and an audio recorder. In the corner of the room, a video camera. Next to the video camera sat a young Harvard researcher named Charlotte, quietly observing and taking notes.

"It's quite the question," Rosa said.

"*My* greatest fear?" Henry said to Charlotte. "Or *our* greatest fear?"

Rosa and Henry didn't think of themselves as particularly interesting subjects for a study. They'd both grown up poor, married in their 20s, and raised five kids together. They'd lived through the Great Depression and plenty of hard times, sure, but that was no different from anyone else they knew. So they never understood why Harvard researchers were interested in the first place, let alone why they were still interested, still calling, still sending questionnaires, and occasionally still flying across the country to visit.

Henry was only 14 years old and living in Boston's West End, in a tenement with no running water, when researchers from the Study first knocked on his family's door and asked his perplexed parents if they could make a record of his life. The Study was in full swing when he married Rosa in August of 1954—the records show that when she said yes to his proposal, Henry couldn't believe his luck—and now here they were in October of 2004, two months after their fiftieth wedding anniversary. Rosa had been asked to participate more directly in the Study in 2002. *It's about time*, she said. Harvard had been tracking Henry year after year since 1941. Rosa often said she thought it was odd that he still agreed to be involved as an older man, because he was so private otherwise. But Henry said he felt a sense of duty to participate and had also developed an appreciation for the process because it gave him perspective on things. So, for sixty-three years he had opened his life to the research team. In fact, he'd told them so much about himself, and for so long, that he couldn't even remember what they did and didn't know. But he assumed they knew everything, including certain things he'd never told anyone but Rosa, because whenever they asked a question he did his best to tell them the truth.

And they asked a lot of questions.

"Mr. Keane was clearly flattered that I had come to Grand Rapids to interview them," Charlotte would write in her field notes, "and this set a friendly atmosphere for the interview. I found him to be a cooperative and interested person. He was thoughtful about each answer, and often paused for a few moments before he responded. He was friendly though, and I felt that he was like the stereotype of the quiet man from Michigan."

Charlotte was there for a two-day visit to interview the Keanes and administer a survey—a very long survey—of questions about their health, their individual lives, and their life together. Like most of our young researchers embarking on new careers, Charlotte had her own questions about what makes a good life and about how her current choices might affect her future. Was it possible that insights about her own life could be locked away in the lives of others? The only way to find out was to ask questions, and to be deeply attentive to every person she interviewed. What was important to this particular individual? What gave their days meaning? What had they learned from their experiences? What did they regret? Every interview presented Charlotte with new opportunities to connect with a person whose life was further along than her own, and who came from different circumstances and a different moment in history.

Today she would interview Henry and Rosa together, administer the survey, and then videotape them talking together about their greatest fears. She would also interview them separately in what we call "attachment interviews." Back in Boston the videotapes and interview transcripts would be studied so that the way Henry and Rosa talked about each other, their nonverbal cues, and many other bits of information could be coded into data on the nature of their bond—data that would become part of their files and one small but important piece of a giant dataset on what a lived life is actually like.

What is your greatest fear? Charlotte had already recorded their individual answers to this question in separate interviews, but now it was time to discuss the question with each other.

The discussion went like this:

"I like the hard questions in a certain way," Rosa said.

"Well good," Henry said. "You go first."

Rosa was quiet for a moment and then told Henry her greatest fear was that he might develop a serious health condition, or that she would have another stroke. Henry agreed that those were scary possibilities. But, he said, they were getting to a point now where something like that was probably inevitable. They spoke at length about how a serious illness might affect their adult children's lives, and each other. Eventually Rosa admitted that there was only so much a person could anticipate, and there was no use in getting upset before it happened.

"Is there another question?" Henry asked Charlotte.

"What's your greatest fear, Hank?" Rosa said.

"I was hoping you would forget to ask me," Henry said, and they laughed. Henry poured more tea for Rosa, took another Oreo for himself, and then was quiet for some time.

"It's not a hard one to answer," he said. "It's just not something I like to think about, to be honest."

"Well they sent this poor girl all the way from Boston, so you better answer."

"It's ugly, I guess," he said, his voice wavering.

"Go ahead."

"That I won't die first is my fear. That I'll be left here without you."

At the corner of Bulfinch Triangle in Boston's West End, not far from where Henry Keane lived as a child, the Lockhart Building overlooks the noisy convergence of Merrimac and Causeway Streets. In the early twentieth century this stubborn brick structure was a furniture factory, and employed men and women from Henry's neighborhood. Now it's home to medical offices, a local pizzeria, and a donut shop. It's also home to the researchers and the records of the Harvard Study of Adult Development, the longest study of adult life ever conducted.

Nestled near the back of a file drawer labeled "KA–KE" are Henry's and Rosa's files. Inside we find the yellowed pages, crumbling at the edges, of Henry's 1941 intake interview. It is written in longhand, in the interviewer's flowing, practiced cursive. We see that his family was among the poorest in Boston, that at age 14 Henry was seen as a "stable, well-controlled" adolescent, with "a logical regard for his future." We can see that as a young adult he was very close to his mother, but resented his father, whose alcoholism forced Henry to be the primary breadwinner. In one particularly damaging incident when Henry was in his 20s, his father told Henry's new fiancée that her $300 engagement ring had deprived the family of needed money. Fearing she would never escape his family, his fiancée called off the engagement.

In 1953 Henry broke free of his father when he got a job with General Motors and moved to Willow Run, Michigan. There he met Rosa, a Danish immigrant and one of nine children. One year later they were married and would go on to have five children of their own. "Plenty, but not enough," in Rosa's opinion.

Over the next decade Henry and Rosa would experience some difficult times. In 1959 their five-year-old son, Robert, contracted polio, a challenge that tested their marriage and caused a great deal of pain and worry in the family. Henry began at GM on the factory floor as an assembler, but after missing work due to Robert's illness he was demoted, then laid off, and at one point found himself unemployed with three children to care for. To make ends meet, Rosa began working for the city of Willow Run, in the payroll department. While the job was initially a stopgap for the family, Rosa became much loved by her coworkers, and she worked full-time there for the next thirty years, developing relationships with people she came to think of as her second family. After being laid off Henry changed careers three times, finally returning to GM in 1963, and working his way up to floor supervisor. Shortly after, he reconnected with his father (who had managed to overcome his addiction to alcohol) and forgave him.

Henry and Rosa's daughter, Peggy, now in her 50s, is also a participant in the Study. Peggy does not know what her parents have shared with the Study because we do not want to bias her reports about her family life. Having multiple perspectives on the same family environment and the same events helps broaden and deepen the Study's data. When we dig into Peggy's file, we learn that when she was growing up, she felt her parents understood her problems, and that they helped cheer her up when she was upset. In general, she saw her parents as "very affectionate." And consistent with Henry's and Rosa's own reports about their marriage, Peggy said that her parents never considered separation or divorce.

In 1977, at age 50, Henry rated his life this way:

Enjoyment of marriage: EXCELLENT
Mood over the past year: EXCELLENT
Physical health over the past 2 years: EXCELLENT.

But we don't determine Henry's health and happiness, or anyone's in the Study, simply by asking them and their loved ones how they feel. Study participants allow us to look at their well-being through many different lenses, including everything from brain scans to blood tests to videotapes of them talking about their deepest concerns. We take samples of their hair to measure stress hormones, we ask them to describe their biggest worries and their critical goals in life, and we measure how quickly their heart rates calm down after we challenge them with brain teasers. This information gives us a deeper and fuller measurement of how someone is doing in their life.

Henry was a shy man, but he devoted himself to his closest relationships, in particular to his connection with Rosa and his children, and these connections provided him with a deep sense of security. He also employed certain powerful coping mechanisms that we will discuss in the coming pages. Building on this combination of emotional security and effective coping, Henry could report over and over again that he was "happy" or "very happy," even during his hardest times, and his health and longevity reflect that.

In 2009, five years after Charlotte's visit to Henry and Rosa's home, and seventy-one years after his first interview with the Study, Henry's greatest fear came true: Rosa passed away. Less than six weeks later, Henry followed.

But the family legacy continues in their daughter, Peggy. Just recently, she sat down for an interview at our offices in Boston. Since the age of 29 Peggy has been in a happy relationship with her partner, Susan, and now, at age 57, reports no loneliness and good health. She is a respected grade school teacher and an active member of her community. But the path she took to arrive at this happy time in her life is harrowing and courageous, and we'll be returning to her later.

THE INVESTMENT OF A LIFETIME

What was it about Henry and Rosa's approach to life that allowed them to flourish in the face of difficulty? And what makes Henry and Rosa's story, or any of the life stories in the Harvard Study, worth your time and attention?

When it comes to understanding what happens to people as they go through life, pictures of entire lives—of the choices people make and the paths they follow, and how it all works out for them—are almost impossible to get. Most of what we know about human life we know from asking people to remember the past, and memories are full of holes. Just try to remember what you had for dinner last Tuesday, or who you spoke with on this date last year, and you'll get an idea how much of our lives is lost to memory. The more time that passes, the more details we forget, and research shows that the act of *recalling* an event can actually change our memory of it. In short, as a tool for studying past events, the human memory is at its best imprecise, and at its worst, inventive.

But what if we could watch entire lives as they unfold through time? What if we could study people from the time that they were teenagers all the way into old age to see what really matters to a person's health and happiness, and which investments really paid off?

We did that.

For eighty-four years (and counting), the Harvard Study has tracked the same individuals, asking thousands of questions and taking hundreds of measurements to find out what really keeps people healthy and happy. Through all the years of studying these lives, one crucial factor stands out for the consistency and power of its ties to physical health, mental health, and longevity. Contrary to what many people might think, it's not career achievement, or exercise, or a healthy diet. Don't get us wrong; these things matter (a lot). But one thing continuously demonstrates its broad and enduring importance:

Good relationships.

In fact, good relationships are significant enough that if we had to take all eighty-four years of the Harvard Study and boil it down to a single principle for living, one life investment that is supported by similar findings across a wide variety of other studies, it would be this:

Good relationships keep us healthier and happier. Period.

So if you're going to make that one choice, that single decision that could best ensure your own health and happiness, science tells us that your choice should be to cultivate warm relationships. Of all kinds. As we'll show you, it's not a choice that you make only once, but over and over again, second by second, week by week, and year by year. It's a choice that has been found in one study after another to contribute to enduring joy and flourishing lives. But it's not always an easy one to make. As human beings, even with the best intentions, we get in our own way, make mistakes, and get hurt by the people we love. The path to the good life, after all, isn't easy, but successfully navigating its twists and turns is entirely possible. The Harvard Study of Adult Development can point the way.

A TREASURE IN BOSTON'S WEST END

The Harvard Study of Adult Development began in Boston when the United States was fighting its way out of the Great Depression. As New Deal projects like Social Security and unemployment insurance gained momentum, there was a growing interest in understanding what factors made human beings thrive, as opposed to what factors made them fail. This new interest led two unrelated groups of researchers in Boston to initiate research projects closely following two very different groups of boys.

The first was a group of 268 sophomores at Harvard College, selected because they were deemed likely to grow into healthy and well-adjusted men. In the spirit of the time, but well ahead of his contemporaries in the medical community, Arlie Bock, Harvard's new professor of hygiene and chief of Student Health Services, wanted to move away from a research focus on what made people sick to a focus on what made people healthy. At least half of the young men chosen for the study were able to attend Harvard only with the aid of scholarships and by holding down jobs to help pay tuition, and some came from well-to-do families. Some could trace their roots in America to the founding of the country, and 13 percent of them had parents who had immigrated to the U.S.

The second was a group of 456 inner-city Boston boys like Henry Keane, selected for a different reason: they were children who grew up in some of Boston's most troubled families and most disadvantaged neighborhoods, but who, at age 14, had mostly succeeded in avoiding the paths to juvenile delinquency that some of their peers were following. More than 60 percent of these adolescents had at least one parent who immigrated to the U.S., most from poor areas of Eastern and Western Europe and areas in or near the Middle East, such as Greater Syria and Turkey. Their modest roots and immigrant status made them doubly marginalized. Sheldon and Eleanor Glueck, a lawyer and a social worker, respectively, initiated this study in an attempt to understand which life factors prevented delinquency, and these boys had succeeded on that front.

These two studies began separately and with their own aims, but were later merged, and now operate under the same banner.

When they joined their respective studies, all of the inner-city and Harvard participants were interviewed. They were given medical exams. Researchers went to their homes and interviewed their parents. And then these teenagers grew up into adults who entered all walks of life. They became factory workers and lawyers and bricklayers and doctors. Some developed alcoholism. A few developed schizophrenia. Some climbed the social ladder from the bottom all the way to the very top, and some made that journey in the opposite direction.

The founders of the Harvard Study would be shocked and delighted to see that it still continues today, generating unique and important findings they couldn't have imagined. And as the current director (Bob) and associate director (Marc), we are incredibly proud to bring some of these findings to you.

A LENS THAT CAN SEE THROUGH TIME

Human beings are full of surprises and contradictions. We don't always make sense, even (or maybe especially) to ourselves. The Harvard Study gives us a unique and practical tool to see through some of this natural human mystery. Some quick scientific context will help explain why.

Studies of human health and behavior generally come in two flavors: "cross-sectional" and "longitudinal." Cross-sectional studies take a slice out of the world at a given moment and look inside, much the way you might cut into a layer cake to see what it's made of. Most psychological and health studies fall into this category because they are cost efficient to conduct. They take a finite amount of time and have predictable costs. But they have a fundamental limitation, which Bob likes to illustrate with the old joke that if you relied only on cross-sectional surveys, you'd have to conclude that there are people in Miami who are born Cuban and die Jewish. In other words, cross-sectional studies are "snapshots" of life, and can prompt us to see connections between two unconnected things because they omit one crucial variable: time.

Longitudinal studies, on the other hand, are what they sound like. Long. They examine lives *through* time. There are two ways to do this. The first we've already mentioned, and it's the most common: you ask people to remember the past. This is known as a retrospective study.

But as we mentioned, these studies rely on memory. Take Henry and Rosa. During their individual interviews in 2004, Charlotte asked each of them, separately, to describe the first time they met. Rosa recounted how she'd slipped on the ice in front of Henry's truck, how Henry helped her up, and how she later saw him in a restaurant when she was out with some of her friends.

"It was funny, and we had a laugh about it," Rosa said, "because he was wearing two different colors of socks, and I thought, 'Boy he's in bad shape, he needs somebody like me!'"

Henry also remembered Rosa slipping on the ice.

"Then I saw her sitting in a café sometime later," he said, "and she caught me staring at her legs. But I was only looking because she was wearing two different colors of stockings, red and black."

This kind of disagreement among couples is common, and probably familiar to anyone who's been in a long-term relationship. Well, anytime you and your partner disagree about the facts of your life together, you are witnessing the failure of a retrospective study.

The Harvard Study is not *retro*spective, it is *pro*spective. Our participants are asked about their life as it *is*, not as it *was*. As in Henry and Rosa's case, we do sometimes ask about the past in order to study the nature of memory, how events are processed and remembered in the future, but in general we want to know about the present. In this case, we actually know whose version of the socks/stockings story is more correct, because we asked Henry the same question about meeting Rosa the year they got married.

"I was wearing different color socks, and she noticed," he said in 1954. "She wouldn't let that happen today."

Prospective, life-spanning studies like this are exceedingly rare. Participants drop out, change their names, or move without notifying the study. Funding dries up, researchers lose interest. On average, most successful prospective longitudinal studies maintain 30 to 70 percent of their participants. Some of these studies only last several years. By hook and by crook the Harvard Study has maintained an 84 percent participation rate for 84 years, and it's still in good health today.

A LOT OF QUESTIONS. REALLY. A LOT.

Each life story in our longitudinal study is built on a foundation of the participant's health and habits; a map of the physical facts and behaviors of their life, through time. To create a complete story of their health we gather regular information on weight and amount of exercise, smoking and drinking habits, cholesterol levels, surgeries, complications. Their entire health record. We also record other basic facts, like the nature of their employment, their number of close friends, their hobbies and recreational activities. At a deeper level we design questions to probe their subjective experience and the less quantifiable aspects of their lives. We ask about job satisfaction, marital satisfaction, methods of resolving conflicts, the psychological impact of marriages and divorces, childbirths and deaths. We ask about their warmest memories of their mothers and fathers, their emotional bonds (or lack thereof) with siblings. We ask them to describe for us in detail the lowest moments of their lives, and to tell us who, if anyone, they could call if they woke up frightened in the middle of the night.

We study their spiritual beliefs and political preferences, their church attendance and participation in community activities, their goals in life and their sources of worries. Many of our participants went to war, fought and killed and saw their friends killed; we have their firsthand accounts and reflections on these experiences.

Every two years we send lengthy questionnaires that include room for open-ended and personalized responses, every five years we collect complete health records from their doctors, and every fifteen years or so we meet them face-to-face on, say, a porch in Florida, or in a coffee shop in northern Wisconsin. We take notes on how they look and behave, their level of eye contact, their clothes, and their living conditions.

We know who developed alcoholism, and who is in recovery. We know who voted for Reagan, who voted for Nixon, who voted for John Kennedy. In fact, before his records were acquired by the Kennedy Library, we knew who Kennedy voted for, because he was one of our participants.

We've always asked how their children are doing, if they had them. Now we are asking the children themselves—women and men who are baby boomers—and one day we hope to ask their children's children.

We have blood samples, DNA samples, and reams of EKG, fMRI, EEG, and other brain imaging reports. We even have twenty-five actual brains, donated by participants in a final act of generosity.

What we cannot know is how, or even if, these things will be used in future studies. Science, like culture, is ever-evolving, and while most of the data from the Study's past have proven useful, some of the most carefully measured variables early on were studied only because of profoundly flawed assumptions.

In 1938, for example, body type was considered an important predictor of intelligence and even life satisfaction (mesomorphs—or the athletically built—were believed to have advantages in most areas). The shape and protuberances of the skull were thought to signify personality and mental capacities. One of the initial intake questions was, for reasons unknown, "Are you ticklish?" and we continued asking that question for forty years, just in case.

With eight decades of hindsight we now know that these ideas range from vaguely harebrained to downright wrong. It is possible, or even likely, that some of the data we are gathering today will be seen with similar bemusement or misgiving eighty years from today.

The point is that every study is a product of its time and the human beings who conduct it. In the case of the Harvard Study, those human beings were mostly White, middle-aged, educated, heterosexual, and male. Because of cultural biases and the almost entirely White makeup of both the City of Boston and Harvard College in 1938, the Study founders took the convenient route of studying only other White males. It's a common story, one that the Harvard Study must grapple with, even as we work to correct it. And though there are findings that apply *only* to one or both of the groups that began the Study in the 1930s, those narrow findings do not feature in this book. Fortunately, we can now compare the findings of the original Harvard Study sample with our own expanded sample (which includes the wives, sons, and daughters of our original participants) and also with studies that include people with more diverse cultural and economic backgrounds, gender identities, and ethnicities. In the coming pages we will emphasize the findings that other studies corroborate—findings that have been shown to be true for women, for people of color, for those identifying as LGBTQ+, for a full range of socioeconomic groups globally—for all of us. The aim of this book is to offer what we have learned about the human condition, to show you what the Harvard Study has to say about the universal experience of being alive.

Marc has taught at a women's college for over twenty-five years, and each year a new cohort of bright, excited students ask to participate in his research on well-being and how people's lives evolve across time. Ananya, from India, was one of these students. She was interested particularly in the links between adversity and adult well-being. Marc told Ananya about the Harvard Study's rich data on hundreds of people spanning their entire adult lives. But they were male, White, and born more than seven decades before Ananya. She wondered out loud what she could learn from the lives of people so different from her—especially old White men born a long time ago.

Marc suggested she spend the weekend reading through the files of just one participant from the Harvard Study, and then they could talk again the following week. Ananya came to the next meeting full of enthusiasm, and before Marc could even ask, said she wanted to do her research on the men in the Harvard Study. What persuaded her was the richness of the life documented in the files she read. Even though the particulars of this one participant's life were so different from her own in so many ways—he came of age on a different continent, lived life with white rather than brown skin, identified as a man not a woman, never went to college—Ananya saw reflections of herself in his psychological experiences and challenges.

This is a story that has repeated itself almost every year; even more so in the last few years as psychology and the world beyond it have reckoned with serious ongoing disparities related to ethnic and cultural backgrounds. Bob himself experienced a similar hesitation when he was first asked to join the Harvard Study as its new director. He, too, had doubts about the relevance of these lives and the quaintness of some of its research methods. He took a weekend to read through a few of the files and was hooked immediately, just as Ananya was. Just as we hope you will be.

An entire century has passed since our First Generation participants were born, but humans are as complex as always, and the work is never over. As the Harvard Study forges ahead into the next decade, we continue to refine and expand our collection of information with the idea that each piece of data, each personal reflection or in-the-moment feeling, creates a more complete picture of the human condition and may help answer questions in the future that we cannot currently envision. Of course, no picture of a human life can ever be complete.

But we hope you'll come with us as we wade into some of the most elusive questions about human development. For example: Why do relationships seem to be the key to a flourishing life? What factors in early childhood shape physical and mental health in mid and late life? What factors are most strongly associated with longer lifespans? Or with healthy relationships? In short:

WHAT MAKES A GOOD LIFE?

When asked what they want out of life, one thing many people say is that they simply want to "be happy." If he's honest, Bob might answer that question for himself in the same way. It's impossibly vague and yet somehow says it all. Marc would probably take a second and then say, "It's more than that."

But what does happiness mean? What would it look like in your life?

One way to find some answers to this question might be to simply ask people what would make them happy, and then find commonalities. But, as we'll show, one hard truth that we would all do well to accept is that *people are terrible at knowing what is good for them.* We'll get into that later.

More important than how people would answer the question are the unspoken and internalized myths about what makes a happy life. There are many, but chief among these myths is the idea that happiness is something you *achieve.* As if it were an award you could frame and hang on the wall. Or as if it were a destination, and after overcoming all of the obstacles in your way, you will finally arrive there, and then just hang out for the rest of your life.

Of course, it doesn't work that way.

More than two thousand years ago Aristotle used a term that is still in wide use in psychology today: *eudaimonia.* It refers to a state of deep well-being in which a person feels that their life has *meaning* and *purpose.* It is often contrasted with *hedonia* (the origin of the word hedonism), which refers to the fleeting happiness of various pleasures. To put it another way, if hedonic happiness is what you mean when you say you're having a *good time,* then eudaimonic happiness is what we mean when we say *life is good.* It is a sense that, outside of this moment, regardless of how pleasurable or miserable it is, your life is worth something, and valuable to you. It is the kind of well-being that can endure through both the ups and the downs.

Don't worry, we won't be saying "your eudaimonic happiness" over and over. But a quick word about what we will be saying, and what it means.

Some psychologists object to the word "happiness" because it can mean anything from a temporary pleasure to an almost mythical sense of eudaimonic purpose that few in reality manage to reach. So in lieu of happiness, more nuanced terms like "well-being," "wellness," "thriving," and "flourishing" have become common in the popular psychological literature. We use those terms in this book. Marc is particularly fond of the terms *thriving* and *flourishing* because they refer to an active and constant state of becoming, rather than just a mood. But we still use "happiness" at times for the simple reason that this is how people talk about their lives. Nobody says, "How's your human flourishing?" We say, "Are you happy?" And it's how, in casual conversation, we both find ourselves talking about our research as well. We talk about health and happiness, meaning and purpose. But we mean eudaimonic happiness. And despite the uncertainty about the word, when people stop to think about what it really means, it's a natural term. When a couple describe their new grandchild and say, "We're very happy," or when someone in therapy describes her marriage as "unhappy," it's clear the word refers to an enduring quality of life, not just a passing feeling. That is the spirit in which we use the term in this book.

FROM THE DATA TO YOUR DAILY LIFE

You might be wondering how we can be so sure that relationships play such a central role in our health and happiness. How is it possible to separate relationships from economic considerations, from good or bad luck, from difficult childhoods, or from any of the other important circumstances that affect how we feel from day to day? Is it really possible to answer the question, *What makes a good life?*

After studying hundreds of entire lives, we can confirm what all of us already know deep down—that a huge range of factors contribute to a person's happiness. The delicate balance of economic, social, psychological and health contributors is complex and everchanging. Rarely can any single factor be said, with absolute confidence, to *cause* any single result, and people will always surprise you. That said, there really *are* answers to this question. If you look at the same kinds of data repeatedly over time, across large numbers of people and studies, patterns begin to emerge, and *predictors* of human thriving become clear. Among the many predictors of health and happiness, from good diet to exercise to level of income, a life of good relationships stands out for its power and consistency.

The Harvard Study is not the only multidecade longitudinal study of human psychological thriving in the world, and we consistently and deliberately look to other studies to see if findings are robust across different eras and different kinds of people. Each study has its own idiosyncrasies, so replication of findings across multiple studies is scientifically compelling.

A few significant examples of other longitudinal studies that collectively represent tens of thousands of people:

The British Cohort Studies include five large, nationally representative groups born in particular years (beginning with a group of baby boomers born just after World War II and most recently including a group of children born at the start of the current millennium) and have followed them across their entire lives.

The Mills Longitudinal Study has followed a group of women since their high school graduation in 1958.

The Dunedin Multidisciplinary Health and Development Study began studying 91 percent of the children born in a small New Zealand city in 1972 and continues to follow them into middle age (and more recently to follow their children).

The Kauai Longitudinal Study ran for three decades and included all of the children born on the Hawaiian island of Kauai in 1955, most of whom were of Japanese, Filipino, and Hawaiian heritage.

The Chicago Health, Aging, and Social Relations Study (CHASRS), begun in 2002, intensively studied a diverse group of middle-aged men and women for more than a decade.

The Healthy Aging in Neighborhoods of Diversity Across the Life Span (HANDLS) study has been examining the nature and sources of health disparities in thousands of Black and White adults (aged 35–64) in the city of Baltimore since 2004.

Finally, in 1947, the *Student Council Study* began tracking the lives of women and men who were elected student council representatives at Bryn Mawr, Haverford, and Swarthmore colleges. This study was planned in part by researchers who had developed the Harvard Study, and was explicitly designed to capture the experience of women, who were not included in the original Harvard Study sample. It lasted more than three decades, and the original archival materials from that study were recently rediscovered. Because of the Student Council Study's connection with the Harvard Study, you will get to meet some of these women in this book.

All of these studies, as well as our own Harvard Study, bear witness to the importance of human connections. They show that people who are more connected to family, to friends, and to community, are happier and physically healthier than people who are less well connected. People who are more isolated than they want to be find their health declining sooner than people who feel connected to others. Lonely people also live shorter lives. Sadly, this sense of disconnection from others is growing across the world. About one in four Americans report feeling lonely— more than sixty million people. In China, loneliness among older adults has markedly increased in recent years, and Great Britain has appointed a minister of loneliness to address what has become a major public health challenge.

These are our neighbors, our children, ourselves. There are myriad social, economic, and technological reasons for this, but regardless of the causes, the data could not be clearer: the shadow of loneliness and social disconnection haunts our modern "connected" world.

You may be asking right now if anything can actually be done about your own life. Are the qualities that make us social or shy just baked into our personalities? Are we destined to be loved or lonely, destined to be happy or unhappy? Do our childhood experiences define us, forever? We get asked questions like this a lot. Really, most of them boil down to this fear: *Is it too late for me?*

It's something the Harvard Study has worked hard to answer. The previous director of the Study, George Vaillant, spent a considerable amount of his career studying whether the ways that people respond to life challenges—the ways they cope—can change. Thanks to George's work and the work of others, we can say that the answer to that enduring question, *Is it too late for me?* is a definitive NO.

It is never too late. It's true that your genes and your experiences shape the way you see the world, the way you interact with other people, and the way you respond to negative feelings. And it is certainly true that opportunities for economic advancement and basic human dignity are not equally available to all, and some of us are born into positions of significant disadvantage. But your ways of being in the world are not set in stone. It's more like they are set in sand. Your childhood is not your fate. Your natural disposition is not your fate. The neighborhood you grew up in is not your fate. The research shows this clearly. Nothing that has happened in your life precludes you from connecting with others, from thriving, or from being happy. People often think that once you get to adulthood, that's it—your life and your way of living are set. But what we find by looking at the entirety of research into adult development is that this just isn't true. Meaningful change is possible.

We used a particular phrase a moment ago. We talked about people who are more isolated *than they want to be*. We use this phrase for a reason; loneliness is not only about physical separation from others. The number of people you know does not necessarily determine your experience of connectedness or loneliness. Neither do your living arrangements or your marital status. You can be lonely in a crowd, and you can be lonely in a marriage. In fact, we know that high-conflict marriages with little affection can be worse for health than getting divorced.

Instead, it is the quality of your relationships that matters. Simply put, living in the midst of warm relationships is protective of both mind and body.

This is an important concept, the concept of *protection*. Life is hard, and sometimes it comes at you in full attack mode. Warm, connected relationships protect against the slings and arrows of life and of getting old.

Once we had followed the people in the Harvard Study all the way into their 80s, we wanted to look back at them at midlife to see if we could predict who was going to grow into a happy, healthy octogenarian and who wasn't. So we gathered together everything we knew about them at age 50 and found that it wasn't their middle-aged cholesterol levels that predicted how they were going to grow old; it was how satisfied they were in their relationships. *The people who were the most satisfied in their relationships at age 50 were the healthiest (mentally and physically) at age 80.*

As we investigated this connection further, the evidence continued to grow. Our most happily partnered men and women reported, in their 80s, that on the days when they had more physical pain, their mood stayed just as happy. But when people in unhappy relationships reported physical pain, their mood worsened, causing them additional emotional pain as well. Other studies come to similar conclusions about the powerful role of relationships. A few touchstone examples from some of the longitudinal studies mentioned above:

With a cohort of 3,720 Black and White adults (aged 35–64), the Healthy Aging in Neighborhoods of Diversity Across the Life Span (HANDLS) study found that participants who reported receiving more social support also reported less depression.

In the Chicago Health, Aging, and Social Relations Study (CHASRS), a representative study of Chicago residents, participants who were in satisfying relationships reported higher levels of happiness.

In the birth cohort study based in Dunedin, New Zealand, social connections in adolescence predicted well-being in adulthood better than academic achievement.

The list goes on. But of course, science is not the only area of human knowledge that has something to say about the good life. In fact, science is the newcomer.

THE ANCIENTS BEAT US TO IT

The idea that healthy relationships are good for us has been noted by philosophers and religions for millennia. In a certain way, it is remarkable that all through history people trying to understand human life keep coming to very similar conclusions. But it makes sense. Even though our technologies and cultures continue to change—more rapidly now than ever before—fundamental aspects of the human experience endure. When Aristotle developed the idea of eudaimonia, he was drawing on his observations of the world, yes, but also on his own feelings; the same feelings we experience today. When Lao Tzu said more than twenty-four centuries ago "The more you give to others, the greater your abundance" he was noting a paradox that is still with us. They were living at a different time, but their world is still our world. Their wisdom is our inheritance, and we should take advantage of it.

We note these parallels with ancient wisdom to put our science into a broader context and to highlight the eternal significance of these questions and findings. With a few exceptions, science has not been much interested in the ancients, or in received wisdom. Striking out on its own path after the Enlightenment, science has been like the young hero on a quest for knowledge and truth. It may have taken hundreds of years, but in the area of human well-being, we are now approaching a full circle. Scientific knowledge is finally catching up to the ancient wisdom that has survived the test of time.

THE BUMPY PATH OF DISCOVERY

Every day the two of us come to work to tackle the question of what makes a good life. As the years have gone on, some results have surprised us. Things we've assumed to be the case in fact were not. Things we assumed would be false have proven to be true. In the coming chapters, we'll be sharing all of it—or a lot of it—with you.

In the next five chapters we explore the elemental nature of relationships and get specific about how to apply the book's most powerful lessons. We talk about how knowing your perch in life—where you are in the human lifespan—can help you find meaning and happiness from day to day. We discuss the massively important concept of *social fitness* and why it's just as crucial as physical fitness. We explore how curiosity and attention can improve relationships and well-being; and offer some strategies for how to deal with the fact that relationships also pose some of our greatest challenges.

In later chapters, we'll dig into the nitty-gritty of specific types of relationships, from what matters in long-term intimacy, to how early family experience affects well-being and what to do about it, to the oft overlooked opportunities for connection in the workplace, to the surprising benefits of all types of friendships. And through it all we will share the science that these insights came from, and we'll hear from Harvard Study participants about how all of these things have played out in their real lives, in real time, for nearly a century.

As director and associate director, we've focused our lives on the Harvard Study and what it can teach us about happiness. We are blessed (and afflicted) by a fascination with the human condition. Bob is a psychiatrist and psychoanalyst who spends hours every day talking with people about their deepest concerns. In addition to directing the Harvard Study, he teaches young psychiatrists how to do psychotherapy. He's been married for thirty-five years, has two grown sons, and in his off hours spends a lot of time on a meditation cushion practicing and teaching Zen Buddhism. Marc is a clinical psychologist and professor who has been teaching and training new psychologists and researchers for thirty years. He, too, is a practicing therapist and is in a long marriage raising two sons. An avid sports fan, he's often found during his off hours connecting with others on a tennis court (and in his younger days, on a basketball court).

The two of us began our research collaboration and friendship almost thirty years ago. We met at the Massachusetts Mental Health Center, an iconic community organization where we both worked with people struggling with mental illness in a setting of tremendous social and economic disadvantage. Both of us felt called to understand the experiences of people from backgrounds very different from our own, both in our clinical work and in our research on lives through time.

Thirty years later, we find ourselves still friends, still collaborating on research, and doing our best to shepherd the Harvard Study's vast treasure trove of life stories toward its second century. In learning about these individuals and their families, we've also learned, and continue to learn, valuable lessons about ourselves, and how to conduct our own lives. This book is an attempt to share those lessons, and to share the priceless gift the Harvard Study's participants have given the world. After all, they didn't agree to participate merely for the sake of researchers like us. They did it for everyone, everywhere. Their lives form the beating heart of this book.

Already we have seen the results of bringing these insights to the larger world. In the course of our careers with the Study, we've given hundreds of lectures on the findings that we'll share in the coming chapters, and we've marshaled everything we've learned into our Lifespan Research Foundation, a nonprofit dedicated to bringing the wisdom of lifespan development out of academic journals and into tools that people can use to better their lives. Over and over, people have approached us after lectures and workshops to say they feel a great relief hearing what we've learned, because the lessons make something abundantly clear: The good life is not always just out of reach after all. It is not waiting in the distant future after a dreamy career success. It's not set to kick in after you acquire some massive amount of money. The good life is right in front of you, sometimes only an arm's length away. And it starts now.

2

WHY RELATIONSHIPS MATTER

The best ideas aren't hidden in shadowy recesses. They're right in front of us, hidden in plain sight.

Richard Farson and Ralph Keyes

Harvard Study, Day 6 of "8 Days" Questionnaire, 2003

Q: What is the secret to aging well?

A: Happiness, caring. Watch what you're eating. Try to get out and do a little walking or exercise. Have friends. It's so good to have friends.

Harriet Vaughn, Study participant, age 80

Consider the feeling you get when you love someone, or when you know you are loved in return. Think about how you experience it in your body, the sensation of warmth and comfort. Now consider the similar but distinct feeling of connection when a close friend helps you through a hard time. Or the lasting exhilaration when someone you respect says they are proud of you. Think about what it feels like to be moved to tears. Or when you get a small boost of energy sharing a laugh with a coworker. Consider the physical pain of losing someone dear to you. Or even the momentary pleasure of waving at the mail carrier.

These feelings, big and small, are connected to biological processes. Just as our brain responds to the presence of food in our bellies by rewarding us with pleasure sensations, so does it respond to positive contact with others. The brain effectively says to us: *Yes, more of this, please.* Positive interaction tells our bodies that we are safe, reducing our physical arousal and increasing our sense of well-being. By contrast, negative experiences and interactions create a sense that we are in danger and stimulate us to produce stress hormones like adrenaline and cortisol. These hormones are part of a cascade of physical reactions that raise alertness and help us respond to situations of critical importance—the "fight or flight" response. They are a big part of what gives us that *feeling* of stress.

We rely on the signals of these stress hormones and pleasurable sensations, as they guide us through the challenges and opportunities of life. Avoid danger, seek connection.

These reactions to rewarding and threatening situations have a long evolutionary history. Homo sapiens have been walking around the planet for hundreds of thousands of years with these biological guides to living built inside of us. That little ping of joy you get when a baby laughs at your silly expression is biologically linked to the one your distant ancestors got when they made a baby laugh in the year 100,000 BC.

Prehistoric humans were threatened in ways we can hardly conceive of today. They had similar bodies, but primitive technology gave them only minimal protection from the environment and predatory animals, and virtually no remedies for injury or other health problems. A toothache could end in death. They lived short, hard, and probably terrifying lives. And yet they survived. Why?

One important reason is a trait that early Homo sapiens shared with many other successful animal species: their bodies and brains had evolved to encourage cooperation.

They survived because they were social.

The human animal is not much different today, though the project of survival has taken on new meanings and complications. Compared to centuries past, life in the twenty-first century is changing faster than ever before, and many of the threats to our lives are of our own making. Along with challenges related to climate change, growing income inequality, and the vast complications of new communications technologies, we must deal with new threats to our internal states of mind. Loneliness is more pervasive than ever before, and our ancient brains, designed to seek the safety of groups, experience those negative feelings as life-threatening, which leads to stress and sickness. With each year that passes, civilization is presented with new challenges that were unimaginable even fifty years ago. It also presents new choices, which means life paths are now more varied than ever. But regardless of the pace of change and the choices many of us now have, this fact remains: the human animal has evolved to be connected with other humans.

To say that human beings require warm relationships is no touchy-feely idea. It is a hard fact. Scientific studies have told us again and again: human beings need nutrition, we need exercise, we need purpose, and *we need each other.*

We are often asked to summarize the findings of the Harvard Study. People want to know: What is the most important thing we've learned? Both of us are by nature resistant to simple answers so these conversations are often not as short as the questioners might like. But when we really think about the consistent signal that comes through after eighty-four years of study and hundreds of research papers, it is that one simple message:

Positive relationships are essential to human well-being.

We'll go out on a limb and guess that if you're reading this book, you are seeking wisdom or you are at least curious about what makes for a good life. You want a life that has meaning and purpose and joy, and you want to be healthy. If we go a little further out on that limb, we might even guess that you are already *trying,* to the best of your ability, to be happy and healthy. You have some idea of who you are, of your likes and dislikes and emotions and social abilities. Day by day you try to live your best life. And if you're like most of us, you don't always succeed.

Throughout this book, we'll be addressing some of the common reasons why people have a hard time finding happiness and satisfaction in life, but there are a couple of general truths that should be acknowledged right off the bat.

The first is this: the good life may be a central concern for most people, but it is not the central concern of most modern societies. Life today is a haze of competing social, political, and cultural priorities, some of which have very little to do with improving people's lives. The modern world prioritizes many things ahead of the lived experience of human beings.

The second reason is related and even more fundamental: our brains, the most sophisticated and mysterious system in the known universe, often mislead us in our quest for lasting pleasure and satisfaction. We may be capable of extraordinary feats of intellect and creativity, we may have mapped the human genome and walked on the moon, but when it comes to making decisions about our lives, we humans are often bad at knowing what is good for us. Common sense in this area of life is not so sensible. It's very difficult to figure out what really matters.

These two things—the haze of culture and the mistakes we make in forecasting what will make us happy—are woven together and play a role in our lives every single day. Over the course of a life, they exert significant influence. The culture we live in leads us in particular directions, sometimes without our even noticing, and we follow along, outwardly pretending that we know what we're doing, but inwardly in a state of low-grade confusion.

Before we talk some more about the cultural and personal ways we can be led away from the good life, let's look at the lives of two Harvard Study participants who have already been through the entirety of life's gauntlet, and see what their experiences can teach us about what matters, and what doesn't.

THE LUCK OF THE DRAW

In 1946, John Marsden and Leo DeMarco were both at major crossroads in their lives. Both had the good fortune of recently graduating from Harvard, both volunteered to serve in the military during World War II—John could not engage in active duty because of health complications and served stateside, and Leo served in the Navy in the South Pacific. Once the war was over, both were about to step forward into the rest of their lives. They had what most people would consider a leg up (or many legs up): John's family was wealthy, Leo's was upper-middle-class, they were graduates of an elite university, and they were male and White in a society that privileged White men. Not to mention that in the aftermath of the war, a lot of social and economic support was being given to veterans through the federally funded G.I. Bill and in local communities. The good life, it seemed, was waiting for them.

While almost two thirds of the original men in the Harvard Study came from the poorest and most disadvantaged neighborhoods in Boston, the remaining third attended Harvard as undergraduates. Groomed to succeed, every one of these college men should have been a poster child for The Good Life in America. Like John and Leo, some came from well-to-do families, most pursued professional careers and married, and many achieved economic and professional success.

Here we see an example of common sense leading us astray. Many of us naturally assume that the material conditions of people's lives determine their happiness. We assume that people who are less advantaged must be less happy and that people who are more advantaged must be happier. Science tells a more complicated story. When you study the lives of thousands of individuals, patterns emerge that do not always fit with popular conceptions about how things are supposed to go. Individual lives like John's and Leo's offer a look at what really matters.

John had a choice: to stay in Cleveland, work in the office of his father's dry goods franchise, and eventually take it over, or to follow his lifelong dream and go to law school (he'd just been accepted to the University of Chicago law school). He was fortunate to have that choice to make. Looking only at the trappings of his life, many people would think that John was destined for happiness.

He decided to go to law school. John had always been a diligent student, and he kept that up. According to John himself, his success was due more to hard work than any special intelligence. He told the Study that his main motivation was a fear of failure, and he even intentionally avoided dating so as not to be distracted. When he graduated from the University of Chicago, he was near the top of his class and began fielding attractive job offers, eventually settling on a firm that encouraged the kind of public service work he hoped to do. He began consulting for the federal government about the administration of public services, and also taught classes at the University of Chicago. His father, though disappointed that John had left the family business, was also very proud. John was on his way.

Leo, on the other hand, had dreamed of becoming a writer and journalist. He studied history at Harvard, and during the war kept meticulous diaries, thinking that he might use them for a book someday. His experiences in the war convinced him that he was on the right path—he wanted to write about how history affects the lives of ordinary people. But while he was overseas, his father died, and soon after he arrived home his mother was diagnosed with Parkinson's disease. As the oldest of three children, he decided to move back to Burlington, Vermont, to care for and be near her, and soon found himself teaching high school.

Shortly after he started his first teaching job, Leo met Grace, a woman with whom he fell deeply in love. They were married immediately and within a year had their first child. After that, the outlines of his life were mostly set. He continued teaching high school for the next forty years and never pursued his dream of becoming a writer.

We skip ahead twenty-nine years, to February 1975. Both men are 55. John got married at 34 and is now a successful lawyer, making $52,000 per year. Leo is still a high school teacher, making $18,000 per year. One day they receive the same questionnaire in the mail.

Let's imagine John Marsden in his law office, sitting at his desk between appointments, and Leo DeMarco at his desk at Burlington High School, while his ninth grade students are puzzling over a history exam. The two men answer questions about their health, their recent family history, and eventually each of them comes to a set of 180 True/False questions. Among them is this one: ·

```
True or False:
Life has more pain than pleasure.
```

To which John (the lawyer) writes:

True.

And Leo (the teacher) writes:

False.

And this one:

```
True or False:
I often feel starved for affection.
```

To this, John responds:

True.

And Leo responds:

False.

They go on to answer questions about their alcohol use (both have one drink every day), their sleep habits, their political ideas, their religious practices (both attend church every Sunday), and later they come to these two questions:

> Complete the following sentences any way you wish:
> A man feels good when . . .

John:

    . . . he is able to respond to inner drives.

Leo:

    . . . he senses that his family loves him despite everything.

And:

> Being with other people . . .

John:

    . . . is pleasant.

Leo:

    . . . is pleasant (up to a point!).

John Marsden, one of the more professionally successful members of the Study, was also one of the least happy. Like Leo DeMarco he wanted to be close to people, as this last answer shows, and he loved his family, but he consistently reported feelings of disconnection and sadness throughout his life. He struggled in his first marriage and alienated his children. When John remarried at the age of 62, he quickly began to refer to that new relationship as "loveless," though it would last to the end of his life.

Later we'll talk more about John's path to despair, and some of the factors that likely shaped his suffering, but there is one particular feature of John's life that concerns us right now: while John tried hard to make himself happy, he was preoccupied at every stage of his life with himself, and what he referred to as his "inner drives." He began his career hoping to make life better for others, but over time associated his achievements less with helping people and more with professional success. Convinced that his career and his accomplishments would bring him happiness, he was never able to find a path to joy.

Leo DeMarco, on the other hand, thought of himself primarily in relation to others—his family, his school, and his friends appear often in his reports to the Study—and he is generally considered to be one of the Study's happiest men. But when one of Harvard's researchers interviewed Leo in middle age, she wrote, "I came away from our visit with the impression that the subject was, well . . . somewhat ordinary."

However, by his own accounting of things, Leo lived a rich and satisfying life. He wouldn't show up on the evening news and his name was not known beyond his local community, but he had four daughters and a wife who adored him, was remembered fondly by friends, colleagues, and students, and throughout his life rated himself as "very happy" or "extremely happy" on study questionnaires. Unlike John, Leo found his work meaningful specifically because he took pleasure in the benefit that other people derived from his teaching.

It's easy enough now, looking back on these two men's lives, to see the links between what they each believed, the decisions they made, and how their lives unfolded. But why is it so difficult in the moment to make decisions that will benefit our well-being? Why do we so often overlook sources of happiness that are right in front of us? An experiment conducted by researchers at the University of Chicago illuminates one central piece of the puzzle.

STRANGERS ON A TRAIN

Imagine you're on a train. Strangers are seated all around you. You'd like to have the most pleasant possible train ride, and you have a choice: talk to a stranger or keep to yourself. Which do you choose?

We know what most of us do: we keep to ourselves. Who wants to deal with a random stranger? They'll probably talk our ear off. Also, we want to get some work done or just enjoy some music or a podcast.

This kind of prediction about what will make us happy is known in psychology as "affective forecasting." We are constantly making predictions about how all kinds of things in our lives, large and small, will make us feel.

Researchers at the University of Chicago turned their local train into an affective forecasting experiment. They asked commuters to predict which of two scenarios—talking to a stranger or minding your own business—would make for a more positive experience. Then they instructed one group to intentionally connect with a nearby stranger and the other group to remain disconnected. When the ride was over, they asked the commuters how they felt about the train ride.

Before the ride, people overwhelmingly predicted that talking to someone they didn't know would be a bad experience, and that keeping to themselves would be much better. They were forecasting what would make them happy, and what would make them miserable. The actual experience, however, was the opposite of what they expected. When commuters were told to strike up a conversation, most had a positive experience and rated their commute as better than usual, and those who typically worked on the train reported that the trip was no less productive when they talked to a stranger.

There is a lot of research like this suggesting that human beings are bad at affective forecasting. Not just in short-term situations like the train study, but in the long term, too. We seem particularly bad at forecasting the benefits of relationships. A big part of this is the obvious fact that relationships can be messy and unpredictable. This messiness is some of what prompts many of us to prefer being alone. It's not just that we are seeking solitude; it's that we want to avoid the potential mess of connecting with others. But we overestimate that mess and underestimate the beneficial effects of human connection. This is a feature of our decision making in general: we pay a lot of attention to potential costs and downplay or dismiss potential benefits.

This is the situation in which many of us find ourselves. We avoid things that we *think* will make us feel bad and pursue things that we *think* will make us feel good. Our instincts don't always lead us astray, but there are important areas in which they do. Like John Marsden, many of us end up making some pretty big decisions (like which career to pursue) or the same small decisions (like never talking to strangers) over and over, based on faulty thinking that seems perfectly logical. Rarely do we get the opportunity to see the error.

This would all be difficult enough if we lived in a vacuum where no outside forces were affecting our decisions; the problem is compounded when we subject our decision making to the cultural influences we face, which themselves contain some ideas that can get us off track. We are not the only ones forecasting what will make us happy; the culture we live in is also forecasting *for us.*

UNDER THE SPELL OF CULTURE

In his commencement address to Kenyon College in 2005, the writer David Foster Wallace used a parable to point out an indelible truth:

> There are these two young fish swimming along, and they happen to meet an older fish swimming the other way, who nods at them and says, "Morning, boys. How's the water?" And the two young fish swim on for a bit, and then eventually one of them looks over at the other and goes, "What the hell is water?"

Every culture—from the broad culture of a nation down to the culture inside a family—is at least partially invisible to its participants. There are important assumptions, value judgments, and practices that create the water we swim in without our noticing or agreeing to them. We simply find ourselves in this world, and we move forward. These features of culture affect just about everything in our lives, often in positive ways, connecting us to each other and creating identities and meaning. But there is a flip side. Sometimes cultural messages and practices point us in directions *away* from well-being and happiness.

So let's stop for a second, as Wallace was encouraging the graduating students to do, and notice some of the cultural water.

In the 1940s and 1950s, when John, Leo, and the other original participants of the Harvard Study were growing into adults, American culture brimmed with assumptions—as it does today, and as it will tomorrow—about what a good life looks like. These assumptions percolated down into their lives, and more importantly, into their life choices. John, for example, was convinced that pursuing law and becoming a lawyer—a respected profession—would lay the groundwork for his future happiness. The culture he grew up in created the conditions for this belief to seem like a truism.

This is complicated terrain because the things that our respective cultures encourage us to pursue—money, achievement, status, and other things—are rarely complete mirages. Money allows us to acquire important things that we need for well-being; achievements are often satisfying and aiming for them can provide goals that give purpose to our lives, and allow us to move forward into new, exciting realms; and status gives us a certain social respect that can allow us to effect positive change. But money, achievement, and status all have a tendency to overtake other priorities. This, too, is a function of our ancient brains: we focus on what is most visible, and most immediate. The value of relationships is ephemeral and hard to quantify, but money can be counted. Achievements can be listed on a résumé, and social media followers tick up in the right-hand corner of your screen. These countable victories give us small pulses of feeling that we like—pleasing sensations, remnants of those ancient signals. As we go through life we can see it all accumulating, and we pursue these goals without always thinking about *why* we're pursuing them. Soon enough we find ourselves beyond the realm where these culturally approved pursuits affect our lives and other people in positive ways, and into the realm where they become ends in themselves. Here, the pursuits become abstracted, more symbolic than tangible, and the chase for a better life starts to look more like running in circles.

There is a lot to say about all of these objects of desire and their psychological underpinnings, but for the sake of illustration let's take a closer look at one emblematic keystone, a persistent cultural assumption, shared among many cultures all over the world, that is not only old but ancient and shows no signs of going anywhere:

The foundation of a good life is money.

Of course very few people would say it like this with a straight face, but signs of the strength of this belief are evident all around us. We see it in the equation of well-paying jobs with "good" jobs, in the fascination with the ultrawealthy, in the increasingly pragmatic educational system ("You go to school to get a 'better' job"), in the glamorous promises of consumer products, and in many other avenues of life. It is a story so much a part of the cultural water that it survives despite the fact that philosophers, writers, and artists have been warning against the seductions of wealth for thousands of years.

Aristotle, for example, outlined the problem two thousand years ago. "The life of money-making is one undertaken under compulsion," he wrote, "and wealth is evidently not the good we are seeking; for it is merely useful and for the sake of something else."

We might list a hundred similar sentiments, articulated in every era of history ("Money has never made man happy, nor will it."—Ben Franklin, or: "Don't make money your goal. Instead pursue the things you love doing and then do them so well that people can't take their eyes off you."—Maya Angelou). All of these sentiments trickle down and coalesce into that clichéd refrain: Money can't buy happiness.

The idea is so common that it has itself been folded into capitalist cultures all over the world. People tell each other all the time that money isn't the answer, and yet money remains a central object of desire in cultures almost everywhere.

The main reason for this is not much of a mystery. The idea that money buys happiness maintains its allure because every day we see the ways it affects how people live.

In America, income inequality has been increasing for decades and is connected to all kinds of other inequalities, from discrepancies in access to health care to the fact that rich people have shorter commutes to work. The overall effect of money is so significant that people with high incomes can expect to live ten to fifteen years longer than people with low incomes. The men in the Harvard Study are no different; on average, the college men had significantly higher incomes than the Boston inner-city men, and lived 9.1 years longer.

So the idea that money may be a major shaper of happiness is, in some ways, a commonsense observation. And yet it does not reflect the whole truth. To understand the extent to which money affects happiness and well-being, we have to look a bit deeper and ask, as Aristotle was suggesting:

What is the money for?

WHAT WE TALK ABOUT WHEN WE TALK ABOUT MONEY

In 2010 Angus Deaton and Daniel Kahneman at Princeton University tried to quantify the relationship of money to happiness using a year-long Gallup survey that resulted in a massive dataset of 450,000 daily responses from a nationally representative sample of one thousand people.

Deaton and Kahneman showed that in the United States, $75,000 seemed to be a kind of magic number at that time. Once a household income was more than $75,000 per year, which was close to the average family income in the U.S. at the time of the study, the amount of money that people earned showed no clear relationship to daily reports of enjoyment and laughter, which were used as indicators of emotional well-being.

This study finding seems to reinforce the idea that money can't buy happiness, but the other half of the finding was equally as significant: for those making less than $75,000 per year, more income did correlate, modestly, with more happiness.

When money is scarce, and basic needs cannot be met with certainty, life can be incredibly stressful, and in this situation, every dollar matters. Having a basic amount of money allows people to meet those needs, have some control over life, and in many countries affords access to better health care and living conditions.

The study by Deaton and Kahneman is memorable for estimating a dollar amount where happiness plateaus, but the meaning of the study was not new. It is largely consistent with other research that has used different methods and been conducted across multiple countries and cultures that vary in wealth. These studies have paid attention both to how money affects individual happiness and to whether increasing wealth for an entire nation affects the overall happiness of the population. Regardless of their methods and locations, these studies point to a similar conclusion: money matters most at lower levels of income where a dollar, euro, rupee, or yuan is used to provide basic needs and a sense of security. Once you get beyond that threshold, money does not seem to matter much, if at all, when it comes to happiness. As Deaton and Kahneman wrote in their study, "More money does not necessarily buy more happiness, but less money is associated with emotional pain."

At lower levels of income, money brings tangible benefits that are necessary for survival, safety, and a sense of control. But at slightly higher levels of income (and this needn't be $75,000) the meaning of money starts to become somewhat more abstract and becomes about other things, like status and pride.

Maybe none of this comes as a major surprise to you. Maybe for you, money is not about stuff, and not about status, but about freedom. Money has a lot of power in the world, you might think, and the more money I have, the more choice and control I will have.

It's understandable to feel this way. Money is woven deep into the foundations of modern societies. It is tied to achievement, to status, to self-worth, to feelings of freedom and self-determination, to our ability to care for and give joy to our families, to fun. To everything. It's natural that we see it as a central medium through which we interact with the world and pursue so many things in life.

Even Leo DeMarco, the teacher, who built his life around connections with his family and students, was very conscious of money. In addition to his careful retirement savings, he set aside a small amount for many years and used those savings to buy a fishing boat (which his oldest daughter named *Dolores*). That boat featured in all of his children's memories. Leo used money as a means to achieve some satisfying personal ends—ends that connected him to the people he cared about.

However, when money becomes the point, rather than a tool, it joins ranks with other persistent objects of desire that are imbued with importance by the culture around us. Things like fame and career success. Or, as Richard Sennett and Jonathan Cobb framed it in their book *The Hidden Injuries of Class*, "badges of ability." That is, personal merits that are publicly acknowledged.

Some of our happiness also depends on what we see when we look at our neighbors. It is human nature to compare ourselves to others. How big is the gap between the lives we see all around us—in the real world, in entertainment and social media—and what we believe is possible in our own lives? Research has shown that the more we compare ourselves to others—even when the comparison is in our favor—the less happy we are. And the bigger the disparities we see, the greater our unhappiness. So, like many things happiness-related, money's effect on us is simple and it's complicated. But maybe the reason we never find an answer to the question *Can money buy happiness?* is because we're asking the wrong question.

Maybe the right question is: *What actually makes me happy?*

A BOY FROM CHARLESTOWN

When Alan Silva was 14 years old he was in love with the movies. In the summer of 1942, he got a job shining shoes in Thompson Square so that twice a week he could head over to a theater in Charlestown and spend his afternoon with James Cagney or Susan Hayward. He'd go with friends, and when they weren't around, he'd go by himself. He'd see every movie twice, and if it wasn't good, the second time he'd complain to the ticket taker. On the way home he might detour to the Charlestown marina to see who he could find, since he was part of the Community Sailing Club, a local organization that taught kids to sail. If nothing too interesting was happening at the marina he'd head up to Chelsea Street and wait for the right kind of delivery truck to drive by—one with a handrail on the back—so he could sneak up behind and hop a ride back home. But he kept that part a secret. "He doesn't do any truck hopping," his mother told the Harvard Study. "I've warned him about losing legs."

Like most of the Boston kids in the Study, the Silva family lived in poverty. Alan's father was a Portuguese immigrant and worked as a machinist at the Navy Yard, and his income was just enough to keep food on the table. Alan, an excitable, busy kid, was blissfully unaware of the financial stress his parents experienced.

The researcher who interviewed him at 14 described him as "wildly adventurous."

"He comes running in all out of breath," his mother said, "and then he just talks talks talks." She was inclined to allow him some freedom, something her mother-in-law, who lived with them in their three-room apartment, always complained about, since she thought Alan would get into the wrong group, start stealing, and his life would go down the drain.

"I'm not too strict," his mother said. "I let him do what other kids do. It's normal. My mother was too strict and it made me moody. Now I read child psychology books."

In addition to being adventurous, Alan was ambitious. If he wasn't at the movies or sailing or hopping trucks, he was home tinkering with an Erector Set that his father bought him for Christmas. He wanted to learn everything he could about building things. He believed he had control over his life, which also led him to believe something many of the other Boston kids in the Study didn't: that he could go to college.

The two groups of the Harvard Study—the Boston men and the Harvard men—are different in many ways. Taken together, the two reflect some hard realities about the effect of poverty and the differences in life outcomes between the working class and the professional class.

But certain relational advantages retain their power across this socioeconomic divide. In Alan Silva's case, he had a mother who loved him; she advocated for him, believed in him, and supported his aspirations. Thanks in part to her encouragement and support, Alan Silva was one of the few Boston men who went to college. Shortly after graduating with a degree in electrical engineering he was hired by the telephone company and had a long career, retiring at age 56.

At 95, Alan doesn't care for new movies, but he catches some of his old favorites on TV. When we asked him in 2006 what he was most proud of in his life, he did not talk about his career or his college degree:

"We'll be married forty-eight years this year. Children turned out good and grandchildren, too. I'm proud of my family."

Alan's story brings to life the lessons of the Harvard Study on the power of relationships, and it reminds us of an important truth: all of us have a rich mix of things we can't control and things we can. Each of us must find ways to work with the hand we're dealt.

HOW MUCH OF OUR HAPPINESS IS UNDER OUR CONTROL?

> Happiness and freedom begin with a clear understanding of one prin-
> ciple. Some things are within your control. And some things are not.
>
> Epictetus, *Discourses*

Epictetus, another of the great Greek philosophers, was born a slave, so the question of control was personal to him. We don't even know the name his mother gave him; Epictetus is a Greek word meaning "acquired."

When we obsess over things that fall outside of our control, Epictetus said, we make ourselves miserable. So an important project of life is distinguishing which is which.

The theologian Reinhold Niebuhr's "Serenity Prayer" is a modern version of this idea, and while the original version is somewhat different, it is commonly quoted in this way:

> *God, grant me the serenity to accept the things I cannot change,*
> *courage to change the things I can,*
> *and wisdom to know the difference.*

People often think, for understandable reasons, True happiness is beyond reach for me because there is so much that I can't help that is set in stone. I'm not genetically gifted; I'm not extroverted; I endured trauma in my past and am still struggling with it; I'm not privileged in the ways that seem to advantage others in this imbalanced and unfair world.

Lots of things matter in the lottery of life. We may not like it, but there are things we are born *with* or born *into* that affect our well-being and are also beyond our immediate, personal control. Genetics matter. Gender matters. Intelligence. Disability. Sexual orientation. Race. And all of these matter, of course, because of our cultural biases and practices. Black Americans, for example, are one of the least advantaged—if not *the* least advantaged—groups in the United States. On average, Black Americans have less savings, higher rates of incarceration, and poorer health outcomes than any other racial group, all of which contribute to a persistent socioeconomic disadvantage that is difficult to break out of. And as Deaton and Kahneman's study and many others show, socioeconomic status can have an effect on emotional well-being.

This brings us back to the Harvard Study, and an important question about its ethnic makeup: How could the lives of White men like John, Leo, and Henry, men who grew up in America in the middle of the twentieth century, have anything to say about modern women or people of color, about people from entirely different countries, cultures, and backgrounds? Aren't the findings of the Harvard Study only relevant to the demographics of its participants?

When Marc is asked this question, he thinks of a startling and influential paper published in the journal *Science*. The paper sought to determine if there was a link between social connection and the risk of dying at any age, and it looked at both women and men from five studies conducted in five different places around the world.

One of these places was Evans County, Georgia, another was eastern Finland.

There are probably few greater contrasts than the life of a Black woman who grew up in the American South in the 1960s and the life of a White man living on the shore of a frozen lake in Finland. At just about any level of experience you can imagine, one would expect to see some major differences.

All five studies were prospective and longitudinal; like the Harvard Study, they looked at lives as they unfolded over time.

For both men and women, geography and race mattered, as they do in many studies. Individuals in Evans County had the highest mortality rates in the study on average, and those in eastern Finland had the lowest. Within Evans County, Blacks had a higher risk of dying at any point in their lives than Whites did, though that difference was relatively small when compared to the difference between Finland and Evans County. Taken together, these differences are stark and meaningful. But this is only a part of the story. Pulling back a bit more, the data for the men and women in all five locations display a remarkably similar pattern: *people who were more socially connected had less risk of dying at any age.* Whether you were a Black woman in rural Georgia or a White man in Finland, the more connected you were to others, the lower your risk of dying in any given year.

This consistency of findings across different locations and demographic groups is what scientists call "replication," the holy grail of research, and not easy to come by. Just because a scientific study found something interesting does not mean that the matter is settled. Good science requires that findings be replicated. Especially when the object of study is something as complex as human life, it is crucial that we find a consistent signal across many studies, all pointing in a similar direction. Only then can we have confidence that what we're seeing is not a fluke.

More than twenty years after this analysis of five studies, another much larger study cemented the connection between relationships and risk of mortality. Julianne Holt-Lunstad and her colleagues looked at 148 studies conducted in countries all over the world (Canada, Denmark, Germany, China, Japan, Israel, and others) with a combined total of more than 300,000 participants. This analysis echoes the findings of the study highlighted in the article in *Science*: across all age groups, genders, and ethnicities, strong social connections were associated with increased odds of living longer. In fact, Holt-Lunstad and her colleagues quantified the association: incredibly, *social connection increased the likelihood of surviving in any given year by more than 50 percent.* Across all of these studies, the mortality rate of individuals with the fewest ties was between 2.3 (men) and 2.8 (women) times higher than that of individuals with the most ties. These are very large associations, comparable to the effect of smoking on getting cancer. And smoking, in the United States, is considered the leading cause of preventable death.

Holt-Lunstad's study was done in 2010. As time goes on, study after study, including our own, continues to reinforce the connection between good relationships and health, regardless of a person's location, age, ethnicity, or background. Although the life of a poor Italian kid who grew up during the Great Depression in South Boston and the life of a 1940 Harvard graduate who went on to become a senator are quite different from each other—and even more different from a modern woman of color—we all share a common humanity. Like the Holt-Lunstad review, analyses of hundreds of studies tell us that the basic benefits of human connection do not change much from one neighborhood to the next, from one city to the next, from one country to the next, or from one race to the next. It is indisputable that many societies are unequal; there are cultural practices and systemic factors causing significant amounts of inequity and emotional pain. But the capacity of relationships to affect our well-being and health is universal.

As we proceed, we'll focus on identifying what you can do, regardless of the society you live in, or the color of your skin. We will highlight the *malleable factors* that have been shown to affect an individual's quality of life, across many disparate circumstances. Factors that can have an impact on your life and that are under your control.

But what kind of impact? How important are the things we can't change versus the things we can?

We are asked this question a lot, in different forms. One of us will be discussing our research after a talk or in a casual setting and suddenly someone will develop a worried look, and we can almost hear the question before it's asked:

"If my main worry is money and health care, is any of this relevant to me?"

Or: "If I'm shy and have trouble making friends, is the good life out of reach?"

Or as one woman recently asked Bob: "If I had a bad childhood, am I just totally screwed?"

Saying something matters and saying it seals one's fate are two very different things. In science, researchers focus on finding differences between groups. We use the unfortunate words "statistically significant" to note when these differences seem reliable. Very small differences, however, can be statistically significant; so small that they are practically meaningless. So in addition to saying these factors matter, we need to think about how *much* they matter.

SLICING UP THE HAPPINESS PIE

The researcher and psychologist Sonja Lyubomirsky has argued, with compelling evidence, that there are real answers to the question "What makes us happy?" In an analysis that would have made Epictetus proud, she examined the degree to which our level of happiness is changeable.

Building on findings from a large collection of studies, from the happiness of twins raised in different families to the connection of life events with well-being, she sought to discover the mutability of happiness. Previous research suggests that human beings have a "happiness set point," or a baseline level of happiness that is influenced largely by genetics and personality traits. Regardless of how unhappy we feel through one period, or how great we feel through another, we are pulled toward that set point. This is a robust finding that has been discussed in the psychological literature for decades. In general, after something happens that causes us to feel happier or sadder, that boost or dip begins to dissipate, and we return to the *general* level of happiness we've always felt. For example, one year after winning the lottery, those lucky lottery winners are indistinguishable from the rest of us when it comes to happiness.

But if it seems like the happiness set point means that our well-being is set in stone, it's worth pointing out that the glass is half full here—or at least 40 percent full. Lyubomirsky and her colleagues used research data to estimate that our intentional activity counts for a lot when it comes to happiness. Our actions and the choices we make account for about 40 percent of our happiness. That's a sizable chunk that is still within our control.

These findings reveal one of the most essential and hopeful truths about human beings: we are adaptable. We are resilient, industrious, and creative creatures who can survive incredible hardship, laugh our way through tough times, and come out stronger on the other end. But there's another side to this, as the concept of a happiness set point and research about lottery winners shows: we also get used to *better* circumstances. Our emotional well-being cannot improve into infinity. We settle in. We tend to take things for granted. This is a key point in the discussion about money. You might believe that making six figures or landing a new job or upgrading from your old Honda will make you happy, but in short order you will have gotten used to that situation, too, and your brain will move on to the next challenge, the next desire. Not even lottery winners can remain euphoric forever.

This does not point to a flaw in the human character, but to a biological fact: we meet all experiences, positive and negative, on the same psychological and neurological playing field in our brain. Here the science dovetails with a central tenet of Stoicism and Buddhism, as well as many other spiritual traditions: the way we feel in life is determined only in part by what happens around us, and to a great extent by what happens inside of us.

David Foster Wallace, in his Kenyon commencement speech that we quoted earlier, noted what modern Western culture (though it applies to others as well) has done to these mental playing fields we all have, providing us:

> extraordinary wealth and comfort and personal freedom. The freedom to be lords of our tiny skull-sized kingdoms, alone at the center of all creation. This kind of freedom has much to recommend it. But of course there are all different kinds of freedom, and the kind that is most precious you will not hear much talked about in the great outside world of winning and achieving and displaying. The really important kind of freedom involves attention, and awareness, and discipline, and effort, and being able truly to care about other people and to sacrifice for them, over and over, in myriad petty little unsexy ways, every day.

THE ENGINE OF A GOOD LIFE

Leo DeMarco, the high school teacher, had four children. Three of them continue to participate in the Study. In 2016 his daughter Katherine visited our offices for an interview and a series of assessments of her physical health and her approach to navigating emotional challenges. During these visits, which typically took about half a day, we asked participants to share memories of a difficult or low moment in their lives. These experiences are illuminating from both a human and a scientific point of view, since low moments are often formative and also give us some indication of how people cope with difficulties. When we asked Katherine to share a low moment, she wrote about the following experience:

> When my husband and I were trying to become parents for the first time, I had four miscarriages in a relatively short period of time. This was probably the first time in my life that I felt that things were out of my control. There is the saying that you learn more from failure than you do from success, and looking back on this time is when I learned that. It tested me and my husband, and I remember being aware that we needed to be on the same page as a couple so the desire for becoming a family did not become all-consuming in our lives. This was a period that brought a lot of sadness to me and my husband. But I also look back to it as a time that we learned to really be a team when the going got tough. We also consciously chose to not let the experience of trying to start a family take over our lives. We had chosen each other as partners and we needed to take care of each other, with or without children.

Relationships are not just essential as stepping-stones to other things, and they are not simply a functional route to health and happiness. They are ends in themselves. Katherine cared deeply about having a child, but she understood that nurturing her marriage was vital and important in and of itself, whether they reached the goal of parenthood together or not. While we try as scientists to quantify their effect on us, relationships are full of rich and constantly shifting momentary experiences, and this is part of what makes them lively antidotes to the repetitions of material life. Other people will always be somewhat elusive and mysterious, and that keeps relationships interesting and worthy of close attention regardless of their immediate utility. "Love by its very nature," the philosopher Hannah Arendt wrote, "is unworldly."

Because of their centrality in our daily experience, relationships are a powerful and pragmatic part of life's puzzle. That pragmatic value has gone underappreciated in modern times. Relationships are the foundation of our lives, intrinsic to everything we do and everything we are. Even things like income and achievement that on first glance seem unconnected to relationships can in practice be hard to separate from them. What would achievement mean if there was no one around to appreciate it? What would income mean if there was no one we could share it with, no social environment to give it meaning?

The engine of a good life is not the self, as John Marsden believed, but rather our connection to others, as Leo DeMarco's life demonstrates. The movements of the engine are those feelings inside us that our ancestors passed down, from the biggest heartbreaks to the subtle sensations of camaraderie to the sadness of loss to the exhilarations of romantic love; or as Jon Kabat-Zinn called it, borrowing a line from *Zorba the Greek*, "the full catastrophe." It's there that the good life happens, in the real-time, momentary experience of connection.

You might be thinking right now, Okay, sure, but how? How do I change my relationships for the better? I can't just snap my fingers. What would change even look like? Where do I start?

Changing your life—especially your habits of daily living—can be challenging. Many of us start out with the best of intentions to improve our lives, only to be overwhelmed by the force of our well-worn mental habits and the momentum of the culture we live in. It's tempting when confronting the complexity of life to say, I've tried, but I just cannot figure this out. I'll just go with the flow.

We see it all the time in our clinical practices. When a person steers in one direction for much of their lives, and that path feels less than full, they find it difficult to open themselves to the possibility that a different, fruitful path actually exists.

Katherine's situation could have easily spiraled downward. She was able to recognize what was outside of her control—whether she could carry a pregnancy to term—and what was within her control—how she could nurture her relationship with her husband. They were able to maintain a close and forgiving relationship throughout this trial in their life. Luckily, Katherine did eventually become pregnant and give birth to a son, whom she referred to as her "Miracle Baby." But even before that final outcome, Katherine had won an important battle. She'd faced a difficult challenge head-on, made good choices about how she would respond to it, and turned her attention toward nurturing the relationship that was most affected and that would help get her through her ordeal.

The lives in the Harvard Study and many other studies tell us that every life takes twists and turns and that the choices we make matter. These lives are evidence that rich possibilities to improve emotional well-being are available at every stage and in every situation of life.

The chapters that follow contain a lot of research and personal stories, and we hope, particularly in these stories, that you will recognize parts of yourself and the people you care about. We also hope that these stories of mistakes and redemption, of both disconnection and love, will encourage you to reflect on the similarities in your own life, to think about areas that are going well for you, and areas that you might like to improve. Each of us has a storehouse of experience to draw on that can point us in the direction of happiness.

We begin with a wide lens, a kind of satellite view of the human lifespan. Locating yourself on this map will help get you started. Because before you can get where you're going, you first have to know where you are.

3

RELATIONSHIPS ON THE WINDING ROAD OF LIFE

Our destiny is frequently met in the very paths we take to avoid it.

Jean de La Fontaine

Harvard Study Questionnaire, 1975

> Can you tell us the life issues that have faced you after
> age 50 that did not seem so important when you were
> younger? How have you tried to master these issues?

As Wes Travers was approaching his 60s, he found himself in a reflective mood. Looking back on his life, he was trying to square his past experiences with the man he was now. How did he get to this place? What events were pivotal? One event in particular kept coming back to him, though he had only the barest memory of it: when he was seven years old his father packed a small bag, walked out the front door of the family's third-floor tenement apartment in the West End of Boston, and never came back. Wes, his mother, and his three siblings had no idea how they would make a living without him, but they also felt a certain relief. When each child was a toddler, their father was gentle and attentive. But as they grew, he changed. He became violent and short-tempered and often brutally beat the older children, sometimes until they bled. He came home drunk in the middle of the night. He was unfaithful to Wes's mother. After he left, a new and welcome peace settled in the home. But so did a new set of struggles and financial responsibilities for the children, who were plunged into adult worries way too soon. His father's absence affected everything about Wes's formative years.

"I wonder what my life would have been like if he'd stuck around," Wes told the Study later. "I don't know if it would have been better or worse, but I think about it."

When the Harvard Study met Wes at the age of 14, his life had already been a long sequence of challenges. His posture was a little stooped, and he suffered from strabismus, a condition that caused one of his eyes to wander. Because of his shyness and difficulty putting his thoughts into words, he struggled to tell the Harvard Study exactly what his life was like, but he managed to provide a basic picture. School was difficult for him. He couldn't focus, he daydreamed, and he got bad grades in just about every subject. When asked, What's your ambition in life? Wes said, "To be a cook."

Like most of us at that age (or really any age), Wes had a hard time seeing beyond his present experience. Overwhelmed by his current troubles, he had no plans and little hope for his future. But the road he would take was not yet decided. If we could go back now and show his teen self what was to come, he would be very surprised how his life turned out. As we'll see, it was not at all as he expected.

THE MAP AND THE TERRITORY

One of the advantages of a lifetime-spanning longitudinal study is that it can be used to map the entire road a person took over the course of their life. This allows events and challenges to be seen in the flow of everything that came before and after. We can trace the lefts and rights, the dead ends, the hills and valleys, and get a sense of the longer journey. Not just what happened, but how one thing may have led to another, and why. There is a storylike quality to these kinds of records. It's hard to read them and not feel something for the participants. Which is as it should be; first and foremost these are records of personal adventures in being human. When these adventures are combined with hundreds of others and translated carefully into numbers, however, they become the raw material of science, revealing not just lives, but patterns of life.

If you were to place your life's timeline alongside the timelines of everyone else reading this book, a set of patterns similar to those of the Harvard Study participants would emerge. Your life would be unique in some of its specifics, as would everyone's, but striking similarities would emerge across gender, culture, ethnicity, sexual orientation, and socioeconomic background. Wes had an abusive father, but for you it might have been tensions in your parents' marriage that left you feeling deep anxiety, or a learning disability that led to bullying and fear at school. These shared human experiences and repeating patterns of life remind us that regardless of how solitary our own struggles and challenges feel in the moment, there are others who have gone through similar things in the past, and others going through them at this very moment. In this way, the outwardly emotionless material of science can have a very moving effect: it can remind us that we are not alone.

And of course, the other thing we all share is the ever-changing nature of our lives, and even of ourselves. Often these changes are so gradual that we can't see them. Our perception is that we are like an unchanging rock in a stream as the world flows around us. But that perception is mistaken. We are forever changing from what we are into what we will be.

This chapter is about taking a bird's-eye view of these patterns, and that winding path of change. Stepping back and considering the big picture illuminates aspects of our own experience—how we are changing and what we can expect—and also what others are going through. Life looks different at age 20 than it does at age 50 or age 80. That old aphorism,

"Where you stand depends on where you sit," is apt. How we see the world depends on our vantage point.

This is a first, basic step that we use as therapists and interviewers when we're getting to know someone. If we sit down with a person, and they are 35, we have a few good guesses about which twists and turns have passed for them, and which might still be ahead. Nobody fits the model perfectly. Life is too interesting for that. But by considering a person's stage in life, we can jump-start the process of understanding their experience. The same effort is useful for any person in your life, and even for yourself. Knowing that you're not alone, that there are predictable challenges that many people face, makes living ever-so-slightly easier.

When we asked Study participants what they thought was most valuable about taking part in an eighty-year study, many of them said that it gave them an opportunity to take stock of their life at regular intervals. Wes was one of these participants. He mentioned more than once that devoting a few moments to reflect on how he felt and what his life was like helped him to appreciate what he already had, and to see what he *wanted*. The good news is that you don't need to be part of a study to do this. It only takes a little effort and a little self-reflection. We hope this chapter will point the way.

YOUR OWN MINI-HARVARD STUDY

If you've ever seen a picture of your mother or father as a young adult, you know how startling it can be. They seem like people we might have met along the road rather than the parents who created us. They often appear less burdened, more carefree, and somehow . . . different. Pictures of ourselves at a younger age can be even more startling. We might look at our younger selves and feel a sweet nostalgia, or maybe a sense of wistfulness, as we're confronted with our physical changes, our abandoned dreams, our once treasured beliefs. For others, like Wes, looking back at a younger age reminds one of sorrows and challenges that are difficult to revisit.

These impressions point to areas of our lives that are important to us, and they can be turned into something helpful using a simple but powerful exercise we developed for our Lifespan Research Foundation (www.lifespanresearch.org). This involves a bit of personal research, but if you're game, come play along.

Find a photograph of yourself when you were about half as old as you are now. If you're under 35, go back to the time you were starting adult life. Really, any photo from when you were a lot younger will do. Don't just imagine that time, try to find an actual photo. The lively reality of a photograph, the details of the place and time, the expression on your face, all help evoke the feelings that make this exercise worthwhile.

Now take a close look at yourself in that photograph. After you stop wondering why you were so into brown clothes, or marveling at your weight or your once luxurious hair, try to place yourself back in the moment when the picture was taken. *Really look*: spend several minutes (a long time!) just taking it in and remembering that era of your life. What were you thinking about back then? What were you worried about? What were you hopeful about? What were your plans? Who were you spending time with? What was most important to you? And perhaps the most difficult question to face: When you think of yourself at that time, what do you regret?

It helps to put your answers to these questions into words. Jot down a few notes, be as detailed as you like. If you have somebody close to you who's curious about this book you're reading, consider asking them to find a photograph of themselves and to do this with you. (As longitudinal researchers, we suggest that if you have a printed photo, consider using it as a bookmark, and when you're finished, leaving it here in this book, along with your notes. Someone you know might get something out of it in the future as they try the exercise themselves; these records of our loved ones' past lives and thoughts are rare, and valuable.)

IN THE FOOTSTEPS OF HISTORY (AND BEYOND)

The Harvard Study is by no means the first effort to extract useful data from lifetimes of human experiences. For millennia people have been trying to unlock the secrets of human life by looking at its patterns, and they have analyzed these patterns in all kinds of ways, often by categorizing them into stages.

The Greeks had various versions of life's stages. Aristotle described three. Hippocrates, seven. By the time Shakespeare wrote about the "seven ages of man" in his famous "all the world's a stage" soliloquy in *As You Like It*, the idea of life happening in stages was likely familiar to his audience. Shakespeare himself probably learned them in grammar school.

Islamic teachings also mention seven stages of existence. Buddhist teachings illustrate the ten stages along the path to enlightenment using the metaphor of ox herding. Hinduism identifies four stages of life, or Ashramas, and these echo many modern psychological life stage theories: *the student*, who learns about the world, *the householder*, who develops a calling and takes care of his or her family, *the retiree*, who retreats from family life, and *the ascetic*, who commits to the pursuit of greater spirituality.

Science has its own perspectives on the biological and psychological development of the human being. But for a very long time, science focused almost entirely on early childhood development. Until recently, psychological textbooks had only short sections on the development of adults. Once someone reached adulthood, the thinking went, that person was fully formed; the only important change was that of decline, both physical and mental.

In the 1960s and 1970s, this perspective began to change. George Vaillant, the director of the Harvard Study from 1972 to 2004, was one of many scientists who began to see adulthood as a period of important flux and opportunity. It's hard to look at the Harvard Study's longitudinal data and come to any other conclusion. There were also new discoveries about the "plasticity" of the human brain showing that decreased brain volume and declining brain function are not the only changes adults experience with age; positive changes also unfold throughout the lifespan.

In short, the most recent science shows that no matter where you are in your life, you are changing, and not just for the worse; *positive* change is possible.

TIMING IS (HALF OF) EVERYTHING

We find two perspectives particularly helpful in making sense of the life cycle. The first, introduced by Erik and Joan Erikson, framed adult development as a series of key challenges that we all face as we grow older. The second is a theory by Bernice Neugarten about the social and cultural expectations around the timing of the events in our lives.

The Eriksons identified life stages based on cognitive, biological, social, and psychological challenges, and they framed these as crises; we either do or we don't meet a particular challenge successfully. And at every point in life we encounter at least one and often more than one of these challenges. For example, in young adulthood we are faced with the challenge of establishing intimacy or becoming isolated. During this period, we find ourselves asking, Will I find someone to love or will I remain alone? In midlife we are faced with the challenge of establishing a sense of generativity or feeling a sense of stagnation (Will I be creative and contribute to the development of the next generation, or will I be stuck in a self-centered rut?). These "Eriksonian" stages have been used by psychologists and therapists for decades to put life's hurdles into a useful context.

Bernice Neugarten, another pioneer in the study of how adults change, has a different take. Rather than defining life completely by a "development clock," Neugarten has argued that society and culture shape development in important ways. Our upbringing and influences (friends, news, social media, movies) create an informal "social clock" or schedule of events that are supposed to occur at specific times in our lives. Social clocks differ from culture to culture, and from generation to generation. Key events like leaving one's childhood home, entering into a committed, long-term relationship, and having children each have their own cultural value and places in the timeline, and we experience these important events as either "on-time" or "off-time," based on whether we think we're meeting society's expectations. Many who identify as LGBTQ+ experience themselves as "off-time," because some of the events used as markers reflect traditional heterosexual lifestyles. Neugarten said that she was herself "off-time" in important ways. She married early and began her professional career late. In her theory, "on-time" events help us feel that our lives are on track, and "off-time" events create worry that we're not on track. We worry not because off-time events are inherently stressful, but because they don't fit others' (and our own) expectations.

These two ideas—life as a sequence of challenges, and variation in the cultural importance of events and their timing—go a long way toward explaining how we feel about ourselves, and how we engage with the world at different points in our lives.

But there is another way to look at the winding road of life: through the lens of our relationships. Because human life is essentially social, when major changes deeply affect us, our relationships are usually a central element of what's in flux. When a teenager moves away from home, what is it that produces most of the powerful feelings involved: living in a new place, or making new friendships and being *away* from parents? When two people marry, is it the ceremony, the event, or the *bond* that changes their lives? As we develop and change over time, it is our relationships that most often reflect back to us who we really are, and how far we've come on our life path.

A good life requires growth and change. This change is not an automatic process that occurs as we age. What we experience, what we endure, and what we do all affect the trajectory of growth. *Relationships are a central player in this growth process.* Other people challenge and enrich us. With new relationships come new expectations, new troubles, new hills to climb, and often we're not "ready." Very few people, for example, are ever perfectly ready to become a parent. But becoming a parent, and being responsible for a tiny human being, has a way of making most of us ready. It pushes us. Somehow we live up to what we have to do, relationship by relationship, stage by stage, and in the process, we change. We grow.

What follows is a short roadmap of these life stages, as seen through the relationships that make them what they are. Compared to the vast literature available on the human life cycle, this is like a map drawn on a napkin. If you find it helpful, you can explore the references we've put in the notes at the back of the book, and take an even deeper dive. You might recognize yourself and some of your own challenges in what follows, and some of it might not apply at all; that's the case for everyone. But even if you don't recognize yourself at every stage, you might recognize people you know and love.

A LIFETIME OF ADULT RELATIONSHIPS: A MINI ROADMAP

ADOLESCENCE (12–19): Walking the Tightrope

Let's start with that infamous life stage, the teenage years. This is a time of rapid growth but also of contradiction and confusion. An adolescent's life burns with intensity as they ascend into adulthood. If we have teenagers in our lives, their path from childhood to adult life can seem precarious— for them and for us. Richard Bromfield captured the feeling of loving a teenager well when he described the "tightropes" that they string for their parents and the people around them. A teenager needs us to:

> Hold but don't baby;
> admire but don't embarrass;
> guide but don't control;
> release but don't abandon.

However unstable this stage might feel to the people around them, it feels even more precarious for teens themselves. They need to accomplish some big tasks as they move toward adulthood, chief among them figuring out their own identity. This involves experimenting with new kinds of relationships and changing existing relationships, sometimes dramatically. Through their encounters with others, teenagers develop new views of themselves, the world, and other people.

From the inside, adolescence feels both exciting and scary. Possibilities abound, but so do anxieties as teenagers find themselves confronted with profound questions like:

- What kind of person am I becoming? Who do I want to be like, and who do I not want to be like?
- What should I do with my life?
- Am I proud of who I am and who I am becoming? How much should I try to be like somebody I respect?
- Will I be able to make my own way in the world? Or will I always depend on the support of others?
- How do I know if my friends really like me? Can I count on them to have my back?
- I'm having intense sexual and romantic feelings and they are blowing my mind. How can I manage this new intensity of intimacy and attraction?

At some point in the teen years, parental figures usually fall off their pedestals and become ordinary (sometimes boring) adults. This creates a temporary vacuum in the role model department. Parental figures remain necessary for support (food, rides, money), but the real action is with friendships, which are exciting, if sometimes volatile, and can involve new levels of connection and intimacy. The question, "Who am I?" is central, and teenagers often find themselves discovering who they are together, trying on new ways of being that include everything from styles of clothing to political beliefs to gender identity. For many people, close friends are never as central as they are when we're teenagers.

From the outside, adolescence can look like a bundle of contradictions. To a middle-aged parent, it may look like *Invasion of the Body Snatchers*—that once adorable and adoring child is now a moody teen who is at one moment childlike and clingy and in the next moment a disdainful know-it-all. The clever title of Anthony Wolf's popular parenting book sums up a parental perspective on this period: *Get Out of My Life, but First Could You Drive Me and Cheryl to the Mall?* Grandparents who watched this transition in their own children might have a different per-spective. To them, this same teenager may represent the joyous future of the world, and the grandchild's shifting sense of self may seem like neces-sary experimentation.

All of these perspectives make sense. Just as the scenery changes on a long road trip, when you look out at the world, what you see depends on where you are in the life cycle. Taking another person's life perspective into account, taking it to heart, is a skill that we can learn. It requires some imagination and some effort, especially in the face of frustration. But it can help us to spend less time complaining and criticizing and wishing that someone else were different, and more time connecting and nurturing.

If you are the parents, grandparents, mentor, teacher, coach, or role model of an adolescent, you might be asking: How can I best support them, even as they seem to want to be independent? What kinds of things can we do to help them emerge from this period stronger and ready for adult life? And how can I survive their adolescence myself?

First, don't be fooled by signals of teenage bravado and claims about self-sufficiency. Teens need you. Some teens will show this by being clingy, but others may insist that they don't need anyone. Of course, they do. In fact, a teen's relationships with adults may be more crucial than at any other time in life. Research tells us that there are advantages for ado-lescents who become more autonomous while still remaining connected to their parents.

One participant in the Student Council Study (the longitudinal re-search linked to the Harvard Study conducted with graduates of three colleges in the Northeast) was able to look back as an adult and see the emotional puzzle of her teen years more clearly. After she'd become a mother of four herself, she reflected on the way her perspective of her mother had changed, and told researchers:

> There is that standard joke of Mark Twain's about how much his fa-
> ther learned between the time the boy was fifteen and twenty. It's that
> way with me and my mother. But of course the change was in me,

not in her. For a long time, I sort of clung. I was very anxious when my mother was around, mainly, I guess, because I was afraid she was going to be living my life for me instead of letting me be myself. Now I sort of realize how perfectly marvelous she is.

Presence matters. The adults an adolescent interacts with as well as the cultural figures in today's saturated media environment provide models for what life is, and what it *can be*. So the availability of in-person, real-time role models is extremely important. Life may be taking place increasingly online (more on that in Chapter Five), but physical presence still really matters. The template for how an adolescent imagines life is heavily influenced by peers, teachers, coaches, parents, the parents of friends (an underappreciated group of role models), and—as in Wes Travers's case—older siblings.

WES'S SIBLINGS STEP UP

Seven years after his father left, Wes Travers became a participant in the Harvard Study, at the age of 14. When asked in what way the kids' father influenced their lives now that he no longer lived with them, Wes's mother said that the children's father had no interest in any of them, and the feeling was mutual. While his absence strained the household in material ways, it also brought the family closer together. In lieu of a father, the children now looked after each other, each contributing to the household income—an average of $13.68 per person, per week—and sometimes chipping in extra to buy one sibling a needed pair of shoes or a coat or a book bag. As the youngest child, and being somewhat meek, Wes had been cared for by the others and protected from having to get a job. They wanted him to go to school instead. In this way, they were remembering themselves at that stage of life—remembering how they felt having to go to work too early in life. They were trying to give Wes the opportunity to have a longer childhood. His older sister, Violet, worked as a nanny and gave Wes spending money to use however he wanted. Each year he looked forward to summer camp, which his older siblings all saved up to pay for. That's what kept him out of trouble, he told the Study, since among the boys he knew, living in Boston in the summertime meant getting into trouble, plain and simple. He looked up to his older brother, a hard worker who, Wes said, "didn't curse in the house" and set a good example for him. An interviewer's handwritten note from the Study's first conversation with the family, in 1945, captures the special place that Wes had in the Travers household:

"Sister Violet said that when Wesley returned home unexpectedly from camp one day, her eyes filled with tears, she was so happy."

But Wes's siblings couldn't protect him forever. When he was 15, only one year after the Harvard Study first visited him, he had to drop out of high school to help support the family. For the next four years he worked as a dishwasher and busboy in various restaurants, had no consistent friends his age, and spent most of his free time at home. His search to be *someone*, to be *something*, had been diverted before it really began. Later he would tell the Study, "Those were hard years. I felt like nothing."

Wes went from being a somewhat sheltered child to being plunged headlong into adult responsibility, working long hours with very little recreation. This meant that he was deprived of many key developmental adolescent experiences. He had to forge his way through days taken up by a menial job, and as happens for many children in challenging circumstances, he had to kick some developmental tasks down the road—tasks like making close friends, figuring out his identity, and learning how to connect with others in more intimate ways. He had a low sense of self-worth and life offered him few opportunities to explore who he was.

Then, when he was 19, the United States entered the Korean War. Unsure of what his life would become, and seeing no future for himself in Boston, Wes did something many of the men in the Harvard Study did: he joined the military. This was both a way out of his adolescence and a way in to friendships with other young men his age from other walks of life—a new experience for Wes. This gave him more of an opportunity to explore new roles and to ponder what he wanted out of life. After what had seemed like an endless period of toil, Wes had entered into a new era of development—his young adulthood.

YOUNG ADULTHOOD (20–40): Weaving Your Own Safety Net

Peggy Keane, Second Generation Study participant, age 53:

> I was 26 years old and engaged to one of the nicest men on the planet. I felt completely adored and loved. As the wedding date grew closer, I felt panicked and knew, in my gut and heart, that I should not be getting married. The truth was, I knew I was gay. The plans and my own fear of that reality prevented me from speaking up. Immediately following the wedding, I quickly began to shut down. I looked for reasons to blame it on my husband, reasons why this marriage would not work. In a matter of months, divorce papers were filed. This whole event is a low point. Not because I came to terms with being gay, but because I caused this incredible man a great deal of pain. I caused my family such grief. I felt completely embarrassed. Again, not about being gay, but for *not figuring out who I was sooner* and for all the grief I caused two families and so many friends who supported our relationship and traveled from so far to celebrate this wedding.

This was a lonely experience for Peggy in the early years of her young adulthood. Her parents, Henry and Rosa, whom we met in Chapter One, were devout Catholics, and this event strained her relationship with them to its limit. She felt lost and isolated.

If adolescence is the first time we begin asking *Who am I?*, then young adulthood is the time potential answers to that question are really put to the test. We typically become more independent from our family of origin, and this means creating new bonds to fill that vacuum. Work and financial independence become central, and the habits we acquire around balancing work and life can stay with us the rest of our lives. Knitting all of this together is the desire and need for intimate attachments that aren't just about romance, but about sharing life and responsibilities with someone we know we can lean on.

From the outside, young adults can appear to members of their family of origin as detached from family relationships as they focus on work and seek to build emotional intimacy with romantic partners as well as families of their own. Parents might look at their children in this stage and mistake this new focus for a lack of caring, or selfishness. Someone in late life might look at a young adult with envy, and maybe even a little pity that young people are overstressed and can't see the beauty and possibilities of the time and choices they have. *Youth is wasted on the young*, as the saying goes.

From the inside, young adulthood can provoke anxiety as we become responsible for ourselves, while at the same time our path in life is uncertain. Young adults can also experience intense feelings of loneliness. For a young adult struggling to find meaningful work, to find friends and a connection to a larger community, or to find love, seeing others succeed in these efforts can be painful.

Young adults often ask themselves questions like:

- Who am I?
- Am I capable of doing what I want with my life?
- Am I on the right path?
- What do I stand for?
- Will I ever find the right person to love? Will anyone love me?

Two of the great sources of excitement in young adulthood—becoming more self-sufficient and getting ahead in the world—can also be traps. To be sure, accomplishing personal goals or career milestones is enlivening and builds confidence, but it's easy to get so wrapped up in the pursuit of achievement that equally enlivening personal relationships fall by the wayside.

The drive for self-sufficiency can turn into social isolation. Close friendships really matter in young adulthood. Even one good friend who understands what we're going through, someone we can confide in and who can help us blow off steam, can make a big difference in our lives. Family still matters, though there's great variation around the world in how young adults relate to their families of origin. In many countries in Asia and Latin America, young adults often continue living with parents until and even after marriage. By contrast, young adults in the United States often find themselves living hundreds or thousands of miles away from their childhood homes. Physical separation isn't necessarily a negative, but keeping parents and siblings in our emotional loop can ease the trials of young adulthood, and give us confidence to take risks.

And finally, romantic relationships and committed intimacy give us a new feeling of home and provide an important haven of confiding and trust.

WES GETS AHEAD IN ONE WAY, FALLS BEHIND IN ANOTHER

When a Harvard Study interviewer tried to contact Wes in his mid-20s, he was nowhere to be found. When the Study caught up to his mother, who was still living in the same Boston tenement, she told the Study interviewer that after serving in the Korean War, Wes was recruited to work in some kind of government organization and was living overseas. The interviewer was, at first, suspicious.

"Mother claims Wes is doing work for the government overseas," the interviewer wrote in his field notes. "Difficult to know if this is something Wes made up to cover his absence, or if he really is working for the government. I would guess the former."

Wes was, in fact, hired by the U.S. government to help train foreign armies after his service in the war, and worked all over the world, from Western Europe to Latin America. He returned from his duties when he was 29 years old with an entirely different perspective on life, culture, and the world in general. According to his sister, Wes "saved every penny" while he was working internationally and was fortunate to have some military benefits and few financial pressures when he came back to the States. He was able to buy a house for his mother, and moved her out of the tenement their family had lived in his entire life.

Wes was handy and capable with house repairs, so he started helping friends and neighbors with various projects for a little extra money.

He was single at that time, dating no one in particular, and told the Study interviewers that he was not inclined to get married. This is an inflection point for many young adults: *Do I want to commit myself to another person? Am I ready?* We know from later records that Wes was feeling nervous about close commitments. He had his parents' difficult marriage in mind, and he'd also watched his older siblings' marriages encounter serious challenges, so he made a conscious decision to avoid romantic attachments. He spent most of his time fixing up the house he'd bought for his mother.

Wes had had a challenging adolescence, but he was now well on his way in the world. He was propelled into adult responsibilities at a young age, joined the military to escape, had lived his 20s entirely in other countries. Now that he was back, he was, in a way, navigating adolescent and early adult challenges he had never fully faced. He pursued things to see if they would be of interest to him; some were, some weren't. He joined a softball team, a woodworking club, and met new friends. To observers he was certainly "off-time" and seemed uncertain of his path in life. But in his own way, he was taking on important developmental tasks and challenges. He was living life at his own pace.

FAILURE TO LAUNCH

As Wes's case shows, the challenges of adolescence don't necessarily end at a certain age. Just because you turn 18 or 25 or even 30 doesn't mean that you are finished with the developmental tasks associated with the teenage years, and that your transition to adulthood is now complete. The effort to make one's own way in the world continues, and some important emotional or career developments can get postponed as other things take priority. This timing is a little different for everyone, and as society changes, the paths through young adulthood have become more and more varied—there are all kinds of possibilities, and all kinds of dangers.

In modern times, particularly in societies that are relatively well-off, there is a kind of extended adolescence that often continues through the 20s. Jeffrey Arnett has labeled this period "emerging adulthood," in which young adults may remain largely dependent on their parents, casting around for their place in the world. The development of some young adults seems to stall during this time, as they never venture very far out from under the wings of their parents.

The path to responsible adulthood has become very complicated, and navigating it is not easy.

In Spain there is a group of young adults called the NiNi generation (*ni estudia, ni trabaja*: "they don't study; they don't work"), who live at home. In the U.K. and other countries, there is an actual public policy designation for this subset of the population: NEETs (not in education, employment, or training).

In Japan, there is the even more concerning phenomenon of *hikiko-mori*, which translates roughly to "pulling inward" or "being confined." This is a slightly different issue, more common in young men than young women, that combines the inactivity of NiNis and NEETs with arrested psychological and social development, an intense social aversion, and sometimes internet addiction through gaming and social media platforms.

In the United States the phenomenon is not so ubiquitous that there is a popular name for it, but young adults do continue to live with parents in considerable numbers and many are struggling to identify a path forward in their lives. In 2015, one third of U.S. adults aged 18–34 lived with their parents, and about one quarter of those, or 2.2 million young adults, were neither attending school nor working.

These young men and women are not living independently, and this can hamper their ability to see themselves as competent adults. A dramatic and compounding effect on intimate relationships often follows as an increasing dependency on parents further stifles the development of self-confidence. But it's not always their fault. The modern economy is unforgiving. Even young adults who go to college and train for a particular profession might emerge with large debts and no assets into an economy that doesn't need them. Parents often provide the safety net.

This is mainly a phenomenon in developed nations and within wealthy groups. By contrast, in developing nations and in less advantaged groups in developed countries, children may begin working and supporting their family at 15 or even younger, just as Wes Travers had done.

COMPETENCY AND INTIMACY

While Wes had delayed some of the tasks of adolescent development into his later years, he was quite far ahead of his peers in establishing competency. He joined the military at 19 and pursued difficult training, earned promotions, and parachuted into enemy territory. This once shy child developed skills as a young adult that bolstered his self-confidence. Normally humble and self-deprecating, he uncharacteristically boasted to the Study at age 34: "You could drop me in any environment anywhere in the world and I believe I could survive, and thrive." When he returned to the States he was unafraid of attempting any hands-on task. He taught himself carpentry and built his own house. The house he bought for his mother and sister with his earnings gave him a feeling of purpose and pride; he was returning some of the care they gave him in the way he knew how.

In general, as young adults we are trying to figure out how to establish ourselves in the two big domains of life—work and family. Some people manage to develop competence in both work and family spheres simultaneously, others flourish more in one sphere.

Finding this balance is a developmental challenge, and the possible solutions have varied across gender. Wes's family is a good example. When he came out of the military, he moved into adulthood with the affection and support of his sister and mother; with this foundation and the right circumstances, his sense of competence blossomed. But in the 1950s and 1960s, the same type of support and encouragement was not available to his sister. Even in the twenty-first century, gender-based norms continue to shape young adult development, both in work and family life. Despite advances, women in many cultures still carry much of the burden of duties around children and the home. This unbalanced division of labor may slow or even hinder young women's development and realization of goals, while allowing men greater freedom to pursue career development.

Although Wes had the support of his sister and mother, he had no significant intimate relationships through his young adulthood. He had come a long way in his sense of competency and control, and he had developed a lot of casual friendships and an active social life. However, the records show some reluctance, uncertainty, and loneliness in Wes's romantic life. He had no one to confide in, no one to share his days with. Although others might not feel the need for romance in their lives, Wes felt the absence of romance as a major void, and he didn't know what to do about it. He could build a house, but he couldn't figure out how to build a home.

MIDLIFE (41–65): Stepping Beyond the Self

1964 Harvard Study Questionnaire for John Marsden, age 43:

Q: Please use the last page(s) to answer all the questions we should have asked, if we'd asked about the things that matter most to you.

A:

1. I'm growing old. Realize for the first time the reality of death.

2. Feel I may not achieve what I wanted.

3. Not sure I know how to bring up children. I thought I did.

4. Tensions at work are severe.

At some point in life we realize that we're no longer young. The generation before us is growing old and we can see (and feel) the beginnings of that same process in our own bodies. If we have children, our roles in their lives are changing as they become their own people, and we worry about what their future will bring. Friendships—so important in adolescence and young adulthood—may take a backseat to responsibilities. We may be proud of our accomplishments and happy with where we are in some ways, and in other ways wish we'd done things differently. Our lives seem to be shedding some of the possibilities they once had. At the same time, we've learned a great deal, and many of us would not choose to go back.

From the outside, the middle years often look stable and predictable. To younger generations, even boring. To older adults looking back, midlife might look like the prime of life—the best mix of wisdom and vitality. These are flip sides of the same perception; when we look at a person in middle age who has steady work, a routine, a partner and a family, we often think, *This person really has it together, they're in control.* Middle-aged adults often look at their peers this way. But the struggles of midlife aren't always visible for others to see.

From the inside, midlife can feel different than it looks. We may have a stable work and home life, and have pride in those things, but also feel more stressed than ever, overwhelmed with responsibilities and worry. Raising children, taking care of aging parents, and juggling the tasks of home and work, middle-aged adults often find neither the opportunity nor the energy to reach out and share their worries with others. The stability and routine that some of us find in midlife will feel like safety and security to one person—*I've established myself and built a life*—but to another like stagnation. We may look at how we got here and wonder if we've chosen the right path (*What would have happened if only . . . ?*). And then of course, as John Marsden's response to the questionnaire above makes clear, at some point we begin to understand on a visceral level that our life is short. In fact, it's probably more than half over. This is a bracing realization, to say the least.

Around the middle of our lives, it's common to ask questions like:

- Am I doing well compared to others?
- Am I in a rut?

- Am I a good partner and parent? Do I have good relationships with my children?
- How many years do I have left?
- Does the life I'm leading have meaning beyond myself?
- What people and purposes do I really care about (and how can I invest in them)?
- What else do I want to do?

Finally, realizing that a lot of life is behind us, we might look around at our lives, see the limits of our abilities and the likely conclusion of the path we are on, and think, *Is this all there is?*

The simple answer is no. There is more. Midlife is an inflection point, not only between young and old, but also between the self-focused, inward-looking way of living that many of us developed in young adulthood and a more generous, outward-looking way of living. This is the most important and enlivening task of midlife: to expand one's focus to the world beyond the self.

In psychology, expanding our concerns and efforts beyond our own lives is called "generativity" and it's a key to unlocking the vibrancy and excitement of midlife. Among Harvard Study participants, the happiest and most satisfied adults were those who managed to turn the question "What can I do for myself?" into "What can I do for the world beyond me?"

John F. Kennedy—himself a Harvard Study participant—came to understand this well in his own midlife. He offered not just political, but emotional and developmental guidance when, as president, he said, famously, "Ask not what your country can do for you, ask what you can do for your country."

When asked at the end of their lives, "What do you wish you'd done less of? What do you wish you'd done more of?" our Study participants, male and female, often referenced their middle years, and regretted having spent so much time worrying and so little time *acting* in a way that made them feel alive:

"I wish I hadn't wasted so much time."

"I wish I hadn't procrastinated so much."

"I wish I hadn't worried so much."

"I wish I'd spent more time with my family."

One participant quipped: "Well I didn't do much of anything so less would be nothing!" Many of these answers were given when participants were in their 70s and 80s, looking back on their lives. But we don't need to wait till then to ask ourselves how we can best spend our time.

Relationships are the vehicle that will allow us both to improve our lives and to build things that will outlive us. If we manage to do this in meaningful ways, the question *Is this all there is?* will be reserved for those times we pull out the last quart of ice cream and it feels far too light.

WES OPENS UP IN HIS MIDDLE YEARS

At 40 Wes Travers had not yet married. In the late 1960s in Boston, this was unusual, or what Bernice Neugarten would have called "off-time." When he was 36 he'd started dating a woman named Amy who was divorced and had a three-year-old son. He helped raise the child, but he and Amy never tied the knot. They now lived together in an apartment in the South End.

Wes had applied to the Boston Police Department, and after several years of waiting for a position, was finally accepted.

This proved to be an extremely positive experience for him. He got along well with his colleagues and was particularly suited to the environment. He now knew people all over Boston, and said he had one of the slower heartbeats on the force, so in any tense situation he thought of his role as the peacekeeper—keeping everyone calm.

When Wes was 44 years old he asked Amy to marry him.

Several years later, when a Study interviewer visited Wes for an interview, she asked him about Amy, and recorded his response in her notes. The passage is worth quoting at length:

Amy, Mr. Travers' wife, is 37 years old and they were married in 1971. She is a Baptist and a college graduate. Mr. Travers described his wife as "great—a terrific person," and indicated that he really meant this; it was not something he was just putting on.

He described the characteristics that most pleased him about his wife as "she is a gentle and compassionate person." He said he likes everything about her; that there is something about her personality that he liked right away that has never gone away. He said she is the kind of person who will be very sympathetic toward those who have less than she does, and mentioned that one of the reasons she had gotten this particular kitten for his birthday last year was that the cat had a scar on its head and one half-missing ear from when it was attacked by a dog. He said that even though she could have chosen a healthy-looking cat, it was just like her to take the one in the litter that had scars like this. He said he is somewhat like that too and he probably would have done the same thing.

He said he could not think of anything that really bothers him about his wife. He said that every once in a while they might have a spat—he does not really know about what—but it is something they just get over in an hour or two, and there have never been any kind of serious disagreements between them. They have never been close to getting a separation or a divorce. In terms of his marriage, he said "it gets better all the time."

In the end, I asked the subject why they had waited so long to get married. He said, "I was afraid I might be a person who was set in my ways—afraid of what I might do to her." He indicated that he did have a certain amount of fear of the intimacy of marriage. However, he now seems to have grown with the marriage and has no such feelings or fears about that anymore.

Wes had avoided a long-term partner his entire adult life, perhaps in no small part because of his early childhood experience of his parents' marriage. This is not unusual. We can develop ideas about ourselves and the world that turn out not to be true. It took him much of his life, but with the help of a loving partner, he overcame this fear, surprising himself, and never looked back.

LATE LIFE (66+): Minding What (and Who) Matters

In a study done in 2003, two groups of participants—one older and one younger—were shown two advertisements for a new camera. Both ads included the same lovely picture of a bird, but the slogans were different.

> **One said:** *Capture those special moments.*
> **The other:** *Capture the unexplored world.*

The participants were asked to choose which advertisement they liked best.

The older group chose the slogan about special moments, the younger group chose the slogan about the unexplored world.

But when researchers primed another group of older people by saying, "Imagine that you'll live twenty years longer than you expect to, and you'll be in good health," that older group chose the ad about "the unexplored world."

This study shows a very basic truth about aging: the amount of time we think we have left on earth shapes our priorities. If we think we have a lot of time, we think more about the future. If we think we have less time, we try to appreciate the present.

In late life, time is suddenly very precious. Faced with the reality of our own mortality, we start asking ourselves questions like:

- How much time do I have left?
- How long will I stay healthy?
- Am I losing it mentally?
- Who do I want to spend this limited time with?

- Have I had a good enough life? What was meaningful? What do I regret?

From the outside, late life is often viewed primarily as a period of physical and mental decline. To the young, old age might look like a distant abstraction; a state so divorced from their experience that they can't even imagine growing old themselves. To someone in midlife, an older person's decline hits a little closer to home and might remind them of their own aging process. In contrast to these notions of decline, the wisdom of older people is often viewed with deep respect and honor, particularly in certain cultures.

From the inside, old age is not so simple. We may be more concerned about time as death approaches, but older folks are also more capable of appreciating that time. The fewer moments we have to look forward to in life, the more valuable they become. Past grievances and preoccupations often dissipate, and what's left is what we have before us. The beauty of a snowy day; the pride we have in our children or in the work we've done; the relationships we cherish. Despite the perception that old people are grumpy and cantankerous, research has shown that human beings are never so happy as in the late years of their lives. We get better at maximizing highs and minimizing lows. We feel less hassled by the little things that go wrong, and we are better at knowing when something is important and when it's not. The value of positive experiences far outweighs the cost of negative experiences, and we prioritize things that bring us joy. In short, we're emotionally wiser, and that wisdom helps us thrive.

But there are still things to learn, still some development ahead, and our relationships are the key to maximizing the joys of late life.

One of the harder things for some people to learn is how to give help, and—even harder for others as they grow older—how to receive help. But this exchange is one of the central developmental tasks in late life. As we age, we become concerned both that we're too needy and that people won't be there for us when we really need them. It's a valid worry. Social isolation is a danger. As work and child care and other time investments wane, relationships that were normally attached to those activities tend to fall away. Good friends and important family connections become more important and should be savored. The sense of limited time makes all of our relationships more important: we have to learn how to balance an awareness of death with staying engaged with life.

THE RESOLUTE COUPLE

When Wes Travers was 79, one of our Study interviewers paid Wes and Amy a visit. She landed in Phoenix in the middle of the afternoon and called Wes. He gave her very specific directions on how to get from the airport to the retirement community, and then from the entrance gate up to their duplex. The directions were clear as day, even a bit overly detailed. As she approached in her car, she realized they must have known the exact travel time from the airport because they were ready for her: she could see the two of them standing in the doorway, waving.

Wes had just come in from his morning walk. Amy offered our interviewer coffee, water, and freshly baked blueberry bread.

Before they settled in to the research tasks at hand—a blood draw for DNA collection and an interview—the interviewer asked the couple about their son, Ryan.

Amy paused, then explained that the family had recently experienced a terrible tragedy: Ryan's wife had been diagnosed with brain cancer the previous year, and died in December. She was only 43. Amy and Wes were just doing whatever they could to help, but Ryan and the kids were all struggling.

"I can't help but think of my family growing up," Wes said. "My dad ran away when I was seven. It changed us. Obviously, he was nothing like Leah, our son's wife—my father was a terrible person. But he left and it changed everything. I worry about that for the kids, how they'll cope. It's hard to be a single parent. For me it was probably good that my father left, I don't know. But for these kids . . . it's going to be hard for them."

TURNING POINTS: A JOURNEY THROUGH THE UNEXPECTED

Let's pause here for a moment to appreciate the unexpected. Lifespan developmental theories often emphasize the predictability and logic of life stages. Yet Wes's life illustrates a truth that we encounter over and over again in the lives of participants in many studies, including the Harvard Study: that the unexpected is perfectly ordinary. Chance encounters and unforeseen events are a big reason why an individual's life can never be completely understood by any "system" of life stages. An individual life is an improvisation in which circumstances and chance help determine the trajectory. While there are common patterns in life, it would be impossible for any person to make it from the beginning to the end of life without an unplanned event sending them in a new direction. There is even some research that suggests that it's these unexpected turns, and not any plan, that most define a person's life and can lead to periods of growth. One wrench thrown into the machine can be more significant than all the gears of planned action combined.

Many of these shocks emerge directly from our relationships. We carry the people we love around with us; they are part of us, and when we lose them or those relationships go awry, the feeling is so visceral that it's almost as if there is a physical hole where that person used to be. But intense change, even of the traumatic kind, presents opportunities for positive growth. Evelyn, one of our Second Generation participants, had an experience in her midlife that is not unusual for either men or women:

> Evelyn, age 49:
>
> My husband and I had started to grow apart, after being together from our college days to the end of our 30s. One evening he said he had something to tell me: he was in love with a woman he met on a business trip. . . . I literally felt the floor had fallen away. . . . The emotional pain I felt for the next year was visceral. It took a huge amount of energy to get up every day, go to work, etc. . . . Eventually we divorced,

he married her, I remarried six years after he first told me. I wouldn't have thought the outcome of this experience would be positive, but it was. My career blossomed, and I met a man who I share a much more full and satisfying life with. I know now I can do well on my own and I have much more compassion and empathy for people who experience loss and rejection. I wouldn't have chosen to go through this experience, but I am glad that I did.

Cultural or even global changes can be similar in their sudden shocks to the system. The Covid-19 pandemic that began in 2020 turned many lives inside out. Economic collapses and wars can do the same. All of the college men in the Harvard Study had plans as the 1940s began, while they were contemplating the end of their college careers. Then Pearl Harbor happened, and every plan, for every student, went out the window—89 percent of the college men fought in the war, and their lives were deeply affected by it. Yet nearly all of the college men reported feeling proud to have served, and many remember it as one of the best and most meaningful times in their lives despite its challenges.

This echoes findings from the longitudinal research project known as the Dunedin Study, which began with 1,037 babies born in New Zealand in 1972–73, and continues today. For a number of the Dunedin participants who struggled in adolescence, military service was seen as an important, positive turning point in their life.

For some generations it was war, for another generation it was the upheaval of the 1960s, or the economic collapse of 2008, or the Covid-19 pandemic. For individuals it might be a tragic accident, a mental health problem, a sudden disease, the death of a loved one. For Wes, it was being abandoned by his father, being forced to drop out of school to go to work, and many other things. The only thing we can expect is that the unexpected—and how we respond to it—will change the course of our lives. In the words of a Yiddish proverb, *Der mentsh trakht, un Got lakht.* Man plans, and God laughs.

And yet, unexpected events are not always challenging. Some are positive twists of fate, and these almost always involve relationships. The people we meet in life are responsible for a huge amount of how our life moves. Life is chaotic, and cultivating good relationships increases the positivity of that chaos and makes the chances of beneficial encounters more likely (more on this in Chapter Ten). Maybe that earlier photo of yourself shows some evidence of positive chance encounters. Nearly every moment of our life does: *If I hadn't taken that class then I would have never met . . . If I hadn't missed the bus that day I wouldn't have run into . . .*

It's true that we can never be in total control of our fate. Just because we're having some good luck doesn't mean we earned it, and just because we're having some bad luck doesn't mean we deserve it. We can't outrun the chaos of life. But the more we nurture positive relationships, the better our chances of surviving and even thriving on this bumpy ride.

WES DRINKS SOME COFFEE AND LOOKS BACK

In 2012, just two years after our researcher's visit, at the age of 81, Wes sat down at his kitchen table with a cup of coffee to answer our biennial questionnaire (there are some faint coffee stains still visible on the pages). Here are a few of his responses:

```
Q#8: Who can you really count on to be dependable when you
need help? Please list all the people you know whom you can
count on in the manner described.
A: Too many to list.

Q#9: What is your relationship like with each of your
children, on a scale from 1 (Negative-hostile and/or
distant) to 7 (Positive-Loving and/or close)
A: 7
```

Q#10: Circle the one dot on the scale that best describes
how often you feel lonely:

(Never)   Some of the time   A lot of the time   All of the time

Q#11:

a. How often do you feel that you lack companionship?

(Hardly Ever)   Some of the time   Often

b. How often do you feel left out?

(Hardly Ever)   Some of the time   Often

c. How often do you feel isolated from others?

(Hardly Ever)   Some of the time   Often

In this questionnaire, he was asked, *What is the most enjoyable activity that you and your wife engage in together?* Wes Travers—who served his country bravely in war, who traveled all over the world, who built his own homes with no formal training, who raised a happy and healthy stepson, and volunteered every day in his community—wrote that the thing he and his wife enjoyed most was: "Just being together."

KEEPING PERSPECTIVE ON THE LIFE CYCLE IN YOUR BACK POCKET

So why bother to think about ourselves in this big-picture way? Can thinking about the process of an entire life really help us from one day to the next?

It can. Sometimes it's difficult to understand and connect with the people in our lives when all we're thinking about is what's right in front of us. Stepping back now and then to take a wider view, to place ourselves and the people we care about into the context of a longer life, is a great way to inject empathy and understanding into our relationships. Some of the frustrations we have with each other can be avoided, and deeper connections made, by remembering that our views of life depend on where we stand in the life cycle.

In the end it's about gaining some perspective on the roads we've taken, and the roads still to come, so that we can help each other anticipate and prepare for the hard curves ahead. And as the old Turkish proverb says, *No road is long with good company.*

4

SOCIAL FITNESS

Keeping Your Relationships
in Good Shape

A sad soul can kill you quicker, far quicker, than a germ.

John Steinbeck, *Travels with Charley*

Harvard Study Second Generation Interview, 2016

Q: Your father participated in the Harvard Study. Looking back on his life, is there anything you learned from him?

A: Dad worked very hard and he was a great engineer but he had a hard time expressing his feelings or even knowing his feelings, so he worked because he didn't know what to do. He played tennis and had friends, but his marriage fell apart, and he tried it with another woman at 66 and it didn't work out. He was 80 and when he died he was alone. And I feel bad for him. I imagine that was true for others of his generation.

Vera Eddings, Second Generation participant, age 55

Psychology often studies the effects of emotional wounds. But we want to talk about one particular study that began by *creating* wounds. Physical ones.

It's not as bad as it sounds; participants had a piece of their skin the size of a pencil eraser removed from their arms just above the elbow, in a procedure known as a punch biopsy. This is a common medical procedure normally used to remove and examine a small piece of skin, but this study was interested not in what was removed but in what was left behind—the wound.

The lead researcher, Janice Kiecolt-Glaser, was investigating psychological stress. She already knew from past research that stress affected the immune system. What she wanted to find out was whether that stress affected other body processes, such as how physical wounds heal.

She sampled two groups of women. The first were the primary caregivers for loved ones with dementia. The second was a group, roughly the same age (early 60s), who were not caregivers.

The study itself was very simple. She performed a punch biopsy on all of the participants, and then watched the wounds heal.

The results were startling. The wounds of the noncaregivers took about forty days to fully heal, but the wounds of the caregivers took nine days longer to heal. The psychological stress of caring for a loved one, which emerged from the slow erasure of important relationships in their lives, was preventing their bodies from healing.

Many years later, Kiecolt-Glaser found herself in the same situation, when her husband and closest research collaborator, Ronald Glaser, developed fast-progressing Alzheimer's disease. When her internist asked her how she was feeling during a regular check-up, Kiecolt-Glaser said she was feeling stressed, and talked about her husband. The internist told her to take care of herself and mentioned that there was now research about stress and health in caregivers—research that Kiecolt-Glaser herself had pioneered. The science had succeeded in making its way into medicine, and back to the source.

THE MIND IS THE BODY IS THE MIND

There is no longer any doubt that the mind and the body are intertwined. When a new emotional or physical stimulus is encountered, the entire mind-body system is affected—sometimes in minuscule ways, sometimes in massive ways—and the changes can have a cyclical effect, with the mind affecting the body, which then affects the mind, and so on.

Modern society, though more medically advanced than ever before, encourages some habits and routines that are not healthy for body or mind. Let's take just one: lack of exercise.

Fifty thousand years ago a Homo sapiens living in a river settlement with her tribe would have gotten the physical exercise she needed simply through the effort of staying alive. Now vast numbers of people are able to provide food, shelter, and safety for themselves with little or no physical exercise. Never before has so much human life taken place in a seated position, and a great deal of the physical work we do is repetitive and potentially damaging. Our bodies do not take care of themselves in this environment—they need maintenance. If those of us in sedentary or repetitive jobs want to maintain our physical fitness, we have to make a conscious effort to move. We have to set time aside to walk, garden, do yoga, run, or go to the gym. We have to overcome the currents of modern life.

The same is true for *social fitness*.

It's not easy to take care of our relationships today, and in fact, we tend to think that once we establish friendships and intimate relationships, they will take care of themselves. But like muscles, neglected relationships atrophy. Our social life is a living system. And it needs exercise.

You don't have to examine scientific findings to recognize that relationships affect you physically. All you have to do is notice the invigoration you feel when you believe someone has really understood you during a good conversation, or notice the tension and distress after an argument, or the lack of sleep during a period of romantic strife.

Knowing how to improve our social fitness, however, isn't easy. Unlike stepping on the scale, taking a quick look in the mirror, or getting readouts for blood pressure and cholesterol, assessing our social fitness requires a bit more sustained self-reflection. A much deeper look in the mirror. It requires stepping back from the crush of modern life, taking stock of our relationships, and being honest with ourselves about where we're devoting our time and whether we are tending to the connections that help us thrive. It can be hard to find the time for this type of reflection, and sometimes it's uncomfortable. But it can yield enormous benefit.

Many of our Harvard Study participants have told us that filling out questionnaires every two years and being interviewed regularly has given them a welcome perspective on their lives and relationships. We ask them to really think about themselves and the people they love, and that process helps some of them. But as we've mentioned, this benefit to them is incidental—a side effect. They have volunteered for research, and our primary focus is learning about their lives. As we move through this chapter, we'll help you develop your own mini–Harvard Study. We've boiled down many of the most useful questions we've asked Study participants into tools that you can use to develop a picture of your social fitness. Unlike the actual Harvard Study, these are not designed to gather information for research. Here, the entire point is to give you the benefit of self-reflection that our Study members received throughout their lives. We began that process in Chapter Three, and this is a chance to go a little bit further.

Looking in the mirror and thinking honestly about where your life stands is a first step in trying to live a good life. Noticing where you are can help put into relief where you would like to be. It's understandable if you have some reservations about this kind of self-reflection. Our Study participants were not always keen on filling out our questionnaires, or eager to consider the larger picture of their lives. (Recall Henry's reluctance to answer the question about his biggest fear.) Some would skip difficult questions, leave entire pages blank, and some would just not return certain surveys. Some even wrote comments in the margins of their questionnaires about what they thought of our requests. "What kinds of questions are these!?" is a response we received occasionally, often from participants who preferred not to think about difficulties in their lives.

The experiences of the people who skipped questions or entire question-naires were also important, though, just as crucial in understanding adult development as the experiences of people eager to share. A lot of useful data and gems of experience were buried in the shadowed corners of their lives. We just had to go through a little extra effort to dig it all out.

One of these people was Sterling Ainsley.

OUR MAN IN MONTANA

Sterling Ainsley was a hopeful guy. A materials scientist, he retired at 63 and thought of his future as bright. As soon as he left his job, he started pursuing personal interests, taking real estate courses and studying Italian on tape. He had business ideas as well, and he began reading entrepreneurial magazines for ideas that fit his interest. When asked to describe his philosophy for getting through hard times, he said, "You try not to let life get to you. You remember your victories and take a positive attitude."

The year was 1986. Our predecessor, George Vaillant, was on a long interview trek, driving through the Rocky Mountains, visiting the Study participants who lived in Colorado, Utah, Idaho, and Montana. Sterling had not returned the most recent survey, and there was some catching up to do. He met George at a hotel in Butte, Montana, to give him a ride to the diner where Sterling wanted to do his scheduled interview (he preferred not to do it in his home). When George buckled himself into the passenger seat of Sterling's car, the seatbelt left a stripe of dust across his chest. "I was left to wonder," he wrote, "the last time somebody had used it."

Sterling had graduated from Harvard in 1944. After college he'd served in the Navy during World War II and then he'd married, moved to Montana, and had three children. For the next forty years he worked on and off in metals manufacturing for various companies across the American West. Now he was 64 and lived on a 50' x 100' grass lot near Butte in a trailer that he could pull behind a truck. He liked having the grass because mowing it was his main form of exercise. He also tended a garden with an enormous patch of strawberries and what he called "the biggest peas you ever saw." He lived in a trailer, he said, because it cost him only $35 a month for hookups, and he didn't feel too committed to the place.

Sterling was still technically married, but his wife lived over ninety miles away in Bozeman, and they hadn't slept in the same room in fifteen years. They spoke only every few months.

When asked why they had not gotten a divorce, he said, "I wouldn't want to do that to the children," even though his son and two daughters were grown and had children of their own. Sterling was proud of his kids and beamed when he spoke of them—his oldest daughter owned a framing shop, his son was a carpenter, and his youngest daughter was a cellist for an orchestra in Naples, Italy. He said his kids were the most important thing in his life, but he seemed to prefer to keep his relationships with them thriving mostly in his imagination. He rarely saw them. George noted that Sterling seemed to be using optimism to push away some of his fears and avoid challenges in his life. Putting a positive spin on every matter and then pushing it out of his mind made it possible for him to believe that nothing was wrong, that he was fine, he was happy, his kids didn't need him.

The previous year his youngest daughter had invited him to visit her in Italy. He decided not to go. "I don't want to be a burden," he said, although he had been learning Italian specifically for that purpose.

His son lived only a few hours away, but they hadn't seen each other in more than a year. "I don't go down there," he said. "I telephone him."

When asked about his grandchildren he said, "I've not gotten too involved with them." They were doing great without him.

Who was his oldest friend?

"Gosh, so many of them died," he said. "So many of them die. I hate to get attached. It hurts too much." He said he had an old pal from out east but hadn't talked to him in years.

Any work friends?

"My friends at work retired. We were good buddies, but they moved away." He talked about his involvement in the VFW (Veterans of Foreign Wars) and the fact he moved up to district commander at one point, but he stepped down in 1968. "It takes a lot out of you."

When did he last talk to his older sister, and how was she doing?

Sterling seemed startled by this question. "My sister?" he said. "You mean Rosalie?"

Yes, the sister he told the Study so much about when he was younger.

Sterling thought about it for a long time, and then told George that it must have been twenty years ago that he last spoke to her. A frightened expression came over his face. "Would she still be living?" he said.

Sterling tried not to think about his relationships, and he was even less inclined to talk about them. This is a common experience. We don't always know why we do things or why we don't do things, and we may not understand what is holding us at a distance from the people in our lives. Taking some time to look in the mirror can help. Sometimes there are needs inside of us that are looking for a voice, a way to get out. They might be things that we have never seen, nor articulated to ourselves.

This seemed to be the case with Sterling. Asked how he spent his evenings, he said he watched TV with an 87-year-old woman who lived in a nearby trailer. Each night he would walk over, and they'd watch TV and talk. Eventually she would fall asleep, and he would help her into bed and wash her dishes and close the shades before walking home. She was the closest thing he had to a confidant.

"I don't know what I'll do if she dies," he said.

LONELINESS HURTS

When you're lonely, it hurts. And we don't mean that metaphorically. It has a physical effect on the body. Loneliness is associated with being more sensitive to pain, suppression of the immune system, diminished brain function, and less effective sleep, making an already lonely person even more tired and irritable. Recent research has shown that for older people loneliness is twice as unhealthy as obesity, and chronic loneliness increases a person's odds of death in any given year by 26 percent. A study in the U.K., the Environmental Risk (E-Risk) Longitudinal Twin Study, recently reported on the connections between loneliness and poorer health and self-care in young adults. This ongoing study includes more than 2,200 people born in England and Wales in 1994 and 1995. When they were 18, the researchers asked them how lonely they were. Those who reported being lonelier were more likely to experience mental health problems, to engage in risky physical health behaviors, and to use more negative strategies to cope with stress. Add to this the fact that a tide of loneliness is flooding through modern societies, and we have a serious problem. Recent stats should make us take notice.

In a study conducted online that sampled 55,000 respondents from across the world, one out of every three people of all ages reported that they often feel lonely. Among these, the loneliest group were 16–24-year-olds, 40 percent of whom reported feeling lonely "often or very often" (more on this phenomenon soon). In the U.K., the economic cost of this loneliness—because lonely people are less productive and more prone to employment turnover—is estimated at more than £2.5 billion (about $3.4 billion) annually and helped lead to the establishment of a U.K. Ministry of Loneliness.

In Japan, 32 percent of adults surveyed before 2020 expected to feel lonely most of the time in the coming year.

In the United States, a 2018 study suggested that three out of four adults felt moderate to high levels of loneliness. As of this writing, the long-term effects of the Covid-19 pandemic, which separated us from each other on a massive scale and left many feeling more isolated than ever, are still being studied. In 2020 it was estimated that 162,000 deaths could be attributed to causes stemming from social isolation.

Alleviating this epidemic of loneliness is difficult because what makes one person feel lonely might have no effect on someone else. We can't rely entirely on easily observed indicators like whether or not one lives alone, because loneliness is a subjective experience. One person might have a significant other and too many friends to count and yet feel lonely, while another person might live alone and have a few close contacts, and yet feel very connected. The objective facts of a person's life are not enough to explain why someone is lonely. Regardless of your race or class or gender, the feeling resides in the difference between the kind of social contact you want and the social contact you actually have. But, then, how can loneliness be so physically harmful when it's a subjective experience?

Answering that question is a bit easier if we understand the biological roots of the problem. As we discussed in Chapter Two, human beings have evolved to be social. The biological processes that encourage social behavior are there to protect us, not to harm us. When we feel isolated, our bodies and brains react in ways that are designed to help us survive that isolation. Fifty thousand years ago, being alone was dangerous. If the Homo sapiens we mentioned earlier was left at her tribe's river settlement by herself, her body and brain would have gone into temporary survival mode. The need to recognize threats would have fallen on her alone, and her stress hormones would have increased and made her more alert. If her family or tribe were away overnight and she had to sleep by herself, her sleep would have been shallower; if a predator was approaching, she would want to know, so she would have been more easily aroused, and she would have experienced more awakenings in the night.

If for some reason she found herself alone for say, a month, rather than a night, these physical processes would continue, morphing into a droning, constant sense of unease, and they would begin to take a toll on her mental and physical health. She would be, as we say, stressed out. She would be lonely.

The same effects of loneliness continue today. The feeling of loneliness is a kind of alarm ringing inside the body. At first, its signals may help us. We need them to alert us to a problem. But imagine living in your house with a fire alarm going off all day, every day, and you start to get a sense of what chronic loneliness is doing behind the scenes to our minds and bodies.

Loneliness is only one piece of the mind-body equation of relationships. It is the visible tip of the social iceberg; much more is submerged beneath the surface. There is now a vast body of research revealing the associations between health and social connection, associations that trace back to the origins of the species, when things were much simpler. Our basic relationship needs are not complicated. We need love, connection, and a feeling of belonging. But we now live in complicated social environments, so *how we meet* those needs is the challenge.

LIFE BY THE NUMBERS

Think for a moment about a relationship you have with a person you cherish but feel like you don't see nearly enough. This needn't be your most significant relationship, just someone who makes you feel energized when you're with them, and who you'd like to see more often. Run through the possible candidates (there may only be one!) and get this person in mind. Now think about the last time you were together and try to re-create in your imagination how they made you feel at the time. Were you optimistic, feeling almost invincible? Did you feel understood? Maybe you were quick to laugh, and the ills in your life and the world felt less daunting.

Now think about how often you see that person. Every day? Once a month? Once a year? Do the math and project how many hours in a single year you think you spend with this person. Write this number down and hang on to it.

For us, Bob and Marc, though we meet up every week by phone or video call, we see each other in person only for a total of about two days (forty-eight hours) every year.

How does this add up for the coming years? When this book comes out, Bob will be 71 years old. Marc will be 60. Let's be (very) generous and say we are both around to celebrate Bob's 100th birthday. At two days per year for twenty-nine years, that's fifty-eight days that we have left to spend together in our lifetimes.

Fifty-eight out of 10,585 days.

Of course, this is assuming a lot of good fortune, and the real number is almost certainly going to be lower.

Try this calculation with your own cherished relationship, or just consider these round numbers: If you're 40, and you see this person once a week for a coffee hour, that's about eighty-seven days before you turn 80. If you see them once a month, it's about twenty days. Once a year, about two days.

Maybe these numbers sound like plenty. But contrast them with the fact that in 2018, the average American spent an astonishing eleven hours every day interacting with media, from television to radio to smartphones. From the age of 40 to the age of 80, that adds up to *eighteen years* of waking life. For someone who is 18, that's twenty-eight years of life before they turn 80.

The point of this mental exercise is not to alarm you. It's to bring clarity to something that goes largely unnoticed: how much time we actually spend with the people we like and love. We don't need to be with all of our good friends *all* the time. In fact, some people who energize us and enhance our lives might do so specifically because we don't see them very often, and like anything else in life, there is a balance that should be struck. Sometimes we are compatible with a person only to a point, and that point is good enough.

But most of us have friends and relatives who energize us and who we don't see enough. Are you spending time with the people you most care about? Is there a relationship in your life that would benefit both of you if you could spend more time together? These untapped resources are often already in our life, waiting. A few adjustments to our most treasured relationships can have real effects on how we feel, and on how we feel about our lives. We might be sitting on a goldmine of vitality that we are not paying attention to—because this source of vitality is eclipsed by the shiny allure of smartphones and TV or pushed to the side by work demands.

TWO CRUCIAL PREDICTORS OF HAPPINESS

In 2008 we telephoned the wives and husbands of Harvard Study couples in their 80s every night for eight nights. We spoke to each partner separately and asked them a series of questions about their days. We mentioned these surveys in Chapter One (they generated a lot of useful data!). We wanted to know how they'd felt physically that day, what kinds of activities they'd been involved in, if they'd needed or received emotional support, and how much time they'd spent with their spouse and with other people.

The simple measure of *time spent with others* proved quite important, because on a day-to-day basis this measurement was clearly linked with happiness. On days when these men and women spent more time in the company of others, they were happier. In particular, the more time they spent with their partners, the more happiness they reported. This was true across *all* couples but especially true for those in satisfying relationships.

Like most older folks, these men and women experienced day-to-day fluctuations in their levels of physical pain and health difficulties. Not surprisingly, their moods were lower on the days when they had more physical pain. But we found that the people who were in more satisfied relationships were buffered somewhat from these ups and downs of mood—their happiness did not decline as much on the days when they had more pain. When they felt worse physically, they did not report declines in mood as much as individuals who were in less satisfying relationships. Their happy marriages protected their moods even on the days when they had more pain.

This might all sound quite intuitive, but there is a very powerful yet simple message nestled in these findings: *the frequency and the quality of our contact with other people are two major predictors of happiness.*

YOUR SOCIAL OBSERVATORY

Sterling Ainsley, so eager to avoid thinking about any of his relationships, believed he was doing pretty well at social fitness. He thought the way he conducted himself with his kids was healthy, he thought his refusal to divorce his wife whom he rarely saw was somewhat heroic, and he even prided himself on his ability to talk with people—a skill he'd developed in his work life. But when asked to look more deeply in the mirror and consider his relationships, it became clear that deep down he felt quite alone, and he had little understanding of how isolated he was.

So where do we start? How can we come closer to seeing the reality of our own social universe?

It's good to start simple. First, ask: *Who is in my life?*

It's a question that most of us, amazingly, never bother to ask ourselves. Even making a basic list of the ten people who populate the center of your social universe can be illuminating. Try it below; you might be surprised at who comes to mind and who doesn't.

WHO ARE MY CLOSEST FRIENDS AND RELATIVES?

_____   _____

_____   _____

_____   _____

_____   _____

_____   _____

A few essential relationships—your family, romantic partner, close friends—probably come to mind quickly, but don't think only of your most "important" or successful connections. List those who affect you from day to day and year to year—good or bad. Your boss or a particular coworker, for example. Even relationships that *seem* insignificant could make the list. We'll talk much more about this in a later chapter, but acquaintances and casual relationships built around activities like knitting, playing soccer, or meeting with a book club could be more important to you than you think. The list might also include people you really enjoy but almost never see: for example, an old friend you often find yourself thinking about but with whom you've fallen out of touch. It might even include people you only exchange pleasantries with, like the driver of the bus you take to work, whom you look forward to seeing and who gives your day a little jolt of good energy.

Once you've got a good set of people, it's time to ask: *What is the character of these relationships?*

We've asked Harvard Study participants a huge variety of questions over the years to try to answer this larger question and create "pictures" (really, datasets) that reflect the character of their social universes. But trying to get some perspective on your own social universe needn't be as complex as research. You can simply think about the *quality* and the *frequency* of contact you have with each person and use two broad dimensions to capture your social world: 1) How a relationship makes you *feel*, and 2) How *often* that happens.

Below you will find a chart that you can use to give your social universe a shape on this two-dimensional spectrum. Where you locate someone on this chart should depend on how energized or depleting that relationship feels, and how frequently you interact with that person. It looks like this:

EXAMPLE OF A SOCIAL UNIVERSE

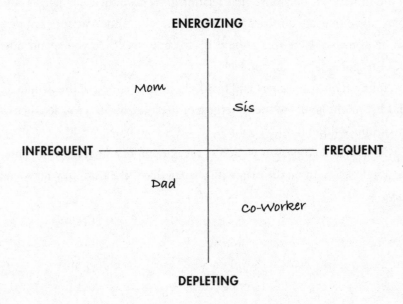

This might seem simplistic at first, . . . and in a way, it is. You're taking something intensely personal and complicated, flattening it, and giving it a static place in this social universe; complexities will be shed in the process. That's okay. This is a first step at capturing the character of the relationships that make your life what it is.

What do we mean by *energizing* and *depleting*?

These are subjective terms, and that's intentional; this is about recognizing how you feel when you are with these individuals. Sometimes we don't really know how we feel about a relationship until we stop to think about it.

In general, an *energizing* relationship enlivens and invigorates you, and it gives you a sense of connection and belonging that remains after the two of you part ways. It makes you feel better than you would feel if you were alone.

A *depleting* relationship induces tension, frustration, or anxiety, and makes you feel worried, or even demoralized. In some ways, it makes you feel lesser or more disconnected than you would feel if you were alone.

This doesn't mean that an energizing relationship will make you feel good all the time or that a depleting relationship will make you feel bad all the time. Even our most vital relationships have their challenges, and many, of course, are a mixed bag. Your general intuition about each person on your list is the thing you want to capture: When you spend time with this person, how do you feel?

Take a look at the chart and think about where each of the people on your list might land. Do they energize or deplete you? Do you see them a lot, or only a little?

That cherished person you don't see enough of can act as your starting point. Set them on the map with a small dot—like a star in your social universe.

MY SOCIAL UNIVERSE

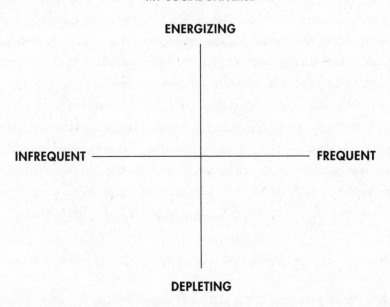

ENERGIZING

INFREQUENT ———————————————— **FREQUENT**

DEPLETING

As you set your relationships in their place, think about each one. Why is this person in this particular place? What is it about the relationship that compelled you to put them there? Is this relationship where you want it to be? If a relationship is particularly difficult and has been giving you a depleted feeling, do any reasons for this come to mind?

Checking in with each relationship like this can help us appreciate and be thankful for people who enrich our lives, and it can help us see which relationships we want to work on improving. Your answers to these questions will (and should) reflect your own preferences about the amount and kind of social connections that suit you. You might realize that you'd like to see *this* person more often, but *that* person is in just the right spot. Maybe *this other* relationship is depleting but important and needs some special attention. If you have a sense of which direction you'd like a relationship to move, draw an arrow from where they are to the spot you'd like them to be.

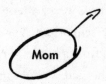

We want to make clear that identifying a relationship as depleting does *not* mean you should cut that person out of your life (although after some reflection you may decide you need to see certain people less often). Instead, it may be a sign that there is something important there that needs your attention. And that means the relationship contains an opportunity.

In truth, almost all relationships contain opportunities; we just have to identify them. Examples include important relationships from our past, positive relationships we have been neglecting, and difficult relationships that may contain the seeds of a better connection. But these opportunities don't last forever; we have to take advantage of them while we can. If we wait too long, we might find, as Sterling Ainsley did, that it's too late.

ROSALIE, HARRIET, AND STERLING

Sterling Ainsley was one of the Harvard College men in the Study, but he was not born into privilege. In fact, he was born directly into his older sister's arms. This was near Pittsburgh, Pennsylvania, in 1923, and Rosalie, his sister, was 12 years old. She'd been home alone with their mother, who was giving Rosalie a French lesson at the kitchen table when she suddenly went into labor. They did not have a telephone and there was no time to fetch the neighbors or a doctor. Through waves of screaming pain their mother managed to give Rosalie instructions about what to do every step of the way, and Rosalie was able to help deliver Sterling safely. She even tied and cut the umbilical cord. "I was extremely close to Sterling," Rosalie told the Study. "As far as I was concerned, I was responsible for him. I treated him like my own child."

Sterling's father was a steelworker and made just enough to support their family of seven, but he was also a compulsive gambler. Every week he would risk his wages, only a fraction of which made it home, so the older kids were forced to work. Three weeks after Sterling was born, his father committed his mother to a sanitarium. For four months, Rosalie took care of Sterling, feeding him from a bottle. "I remember walking the floor with him, singing songs," she said. "When my mother came home, she was different. My father was illiterate, but my mother had been a brilliant woman and spoke three languages with us and taught us how to read and write both English and French, but after that she was never the same. She couldn't take care of Sterling. She didn't know what to do, even though she'd already raised four kids. So I looked after him for several years."

When Sterling was nine years old, his father again committed his mother to a sanitarium, this time permanently, and then abruptly moved away, leaving the younger children to fend for themselves. By this time, Rosalie, at 21 years old, was married and had a child of her own, and she and her husband took three of her siblings into their home. She wanted to bring Sterling also, but a family friend, Harriet Ainsley, had recently lost her own son to a tragic accident and offered to take Sterling and raise him as her own. Already strained financially, Rosalie and her husband agreed.

The Ainsleys lived on a farm in rural Pennsylvania and the lifestyle was a shock for Sterling, but his adoptive parents were kind, calm, and supportive. His adoptive father was stern but fair, and taught Sterling everything he could about how to run and operate the farm. When Sterling was 19 he said of Harriet, his adoptive mother, "She means about everything in the world to me. She has been a wonderful mother. I think she has been responsible for my aspiring to anything. She is the one who gave me a great interest in English literature."

Thanks in part to encouragement from his adoptive mother and his sister Rosalie, Sterling did well in high school, ran (and lost) a campaign for school president, and was accepted to Harvard with a scholarship. When Sterling entered the Study at age 19, Rosalie was asked what she thought of him, and she said, "It's hard to describe him today. He has a tendency, I think, to bring out the best in people that he comes in contact with. He has high ideals. When I spend a day with Sterling, I feel as though I have been to some higher institution of learning."

These two brave and resilient women, Rosalie and Harriet, played pivotal roles in Sterling's life. His biological mother, who was not a part of his life, nonetheless played a vital role through her cultivation of the kindness, caring, and determination in Rosalie that then allowed Rosalie to raise Sterling by herself in those early years. Still, their father was abusive to Sterling, something Rosalie could not control, and the eventual breakup of the family was extremely difficult for Sterling. If it wasn't for each of the women who loved him in turn, it is highly unlikely Sterling would have gone to college and made a life for himself out west. As working-class women in the early half of the twentieth century, there was much preventing them from pursuing their own personal priorities. But they did their best to help Sterling. He said many times in his interviews how grateful he was for their support and for their love.

And yet he lost touch with both of them.

THE KEYSTONES OF RELATIONSHIPS

We've been saying that human beings are social creatures; in essence this simply means that each of us as individuals cannot provide everything we need for ourselves. We can't confide in ourselves, romance ourselves, mentor ourselves, or help ourselves move a sofa. We need others to interact with and to help us, and we flourish when we provide that same connection and support to others. *This process of giving and receiving is the foundation of a meaningful life.* How we feel about our social universe is directly related to the kinds of things we are receiving from and giving to other people. When Study participants expressed a sense of frustration or dissatisfaction with their social lives, as Sterling did in his later life, it could often be traced to a particular kind of support that was missing.

Here are the sorts of questions about various types of support that the Study has asked participants about over the years:

Safety and Security

```
Who would you call if you woke up scared in the middle of
the night?
Who would you turn to in a moment of crisis?
```

Relationships that give us a sense of safety and security are the fundamental building blocks of our relational lives. If you can list specific people in response to the above questions, you are very fortunate—those relationships are crucial to cultivate and appreciate. They help us navigate through times of stress and give us the courage to explore new experiences. What's essential is the conviction that these relationships will be there for us if things go wrong.

Learning and Growth

> Who encourages you to try new things, to take chances, to
> pursue your life's goals?

Feeling secure enough to venture out into unknown territory is one thing, but being encouraged or inspired to do so by someone we trust is a precious gift.

Emotional Closeness and Confiding

> Who knows everything (or most things) about you?
> Who can you call on when you're feeling low and be honest
> with them about how you're feeling?
> Who can you ask for advice (and trust what they say)?

Identity Affirmation and Shared Experience

> Is there someone in your life who has shared many
> experiences with you and who helps strengthen your sense of
> who you are and where you've come from?

Friends from childhood, siblings, people you shared major life experiences with—these relationships are often neglected because they have been with us for so long, but they are especially valuable because they cannot be replaced. As the song goes, *You can't make old friends.*

Romantic Intimacy (Love and Sex)

```
Do you feel satisfied with the amount of romantic intimacy
in your life?
Are you satisfied in your sexual relationships?
```

Romance is something most of us hope for, not only for sexual satisfaction, but also for the intimacy of another's touch, the sharing of day-to-day joys and sorrows, and the meaning that comes with witnessing each other's experiences. For some of us, romantic love feels like an essential part of life. For others, not so much. Marriage, of course, is not necessarily the benchmark of romantic intimacy. The proportion of people ages 25 to 50 who never marry has increased dramatically in the last half century in many places around the world. In the U.S., this proportion increased, from 9 percent in 1970 to 35 percent in 2018. These figures do not tell us the percentage who experience romantic intimacy, but they are an indicator that in the U.S. more people remain unmarried in their adult lives than perhaps ever before. In addition, some committed partnerships are "open," including people outside the couple in both sexual and emotional intimacy.

Help—Both Informational and Practical

```
Who do you turn to if you need some expertise or help
solving a practical problem (e.g., you need to plant
a tree, fix your WiFi connection, apply for health
insurance)?
```

Fun and Relaxation

Who makes you laugh?

Who do you call to see a movie or go on a road trip?

Who makes you feel relaxed, connected, at ease?

Below you'll find a table arranged around these keystones of support. The first column is for the relationships you think have the greatest impact on you. Place a plus (+) symbol in the appropriate columns if a relationship seems to add to that type of support in your life, and a minus (-) symbol if a relationship lacks that type of support. Remember: it's okay if not all (or even most) relationships offer you *all* of these types of support.

SOURCES OF SUPPORT IN MY LIFE

My Relationship With	Safety and Security	Learning and Growth	Emotional Closeness and Confiding	Identity Affirmation and Shared Experience	Romantic Intimacy	Help (Both Info and Practical)	Fun and Relaxation

Think of this exercise like an X-ray—a tool that helps you see below the surface of your social universe. Not all of these types of support will feel important to you, but consider which of them do feel important, and ask yourself if you're getting enough support in those areas. If you're feeling a certain dissatisfaction in your life, do any of the gaps on the chart resonate with that feeling? Maybe you realize you have plenty of people you have fun with, but nobody you can turn to when you need someone to confide in. Or vice versa.

As you fill in and expand this table, you might see some gaps, and also some surprises. You might not have realized that you only have one person you go to for help, or that a person you take for granted actually makes you feel safe and secure, or that another person reinforces your sense of identity in important ways. We know from personal experience (and many conversations over drinks at conferences) that even professionals in the fields of psychology and psychiatry have a hard time seeing their own lives in this way without focused reflection.

MOVING FORWARD

Sometimes this kind of reflection alone will point us in the direction we'd like to go, but even after we see what we'd like to change we may still have trouble taking the first steps.

There is an entire field of research that studies human motivation—why we make the decisions we make, why some people make efforts to change while others never manage it. This research is popular among advertisers, who use it to encourage us to buy stuff. But we can also use it to encourage ourselves to do things we want—like take steps toward growth in our relationships. In fact, we've already applied some of it in this chapter: one of the things this research shows is that a key to motivating change is recognizing the difference between where we are and where we would like to be. Defining these two states creates a kind of potential energy that helps us to take that first difficult step. This is what you have started to do with these relational tools. You've mapped your social universe and the quality of your relationships, and you've reflected on what you might like to change. From here, the process of actually doing it can be messy—particularly for challenging relationships—but the potential rewards are great. We'll get into that process more in coming chapters, but there are a few things you can do immediately, and some useful principles to keep in mind.

WORKING FROM THE TOP DOWN

Focus first on what's working well. This is the easiest place to begin. Take a look at the relationships on the energizing side of your social universe and consider how you might solidify or encourage what's great about them. Tell (and show!) those people how much you appreciate them, and why. It never hurts to double down on what's already bringing energy and vitality into your life. These relationships are already rolling, but there are usually one or two that have slowed down and need a little push to get up and running at full tilt again. Even good relationships tend to repeat the same routines over and over. It might be time to try some new things with them.

Next, take a look at those relationships that are just peeking over that energizing line, or are maybe a little bit depleting on balance. Is there a way you can give these relationships a nudge, and make them more energizing? Minor changes in these relationships can sometimes relieve small burdens that have been adding up.

The relationships you've identified as depleting might require some more consideration and reflection. You might need to take a risk and reach out to someone you might not normally contact, message them, plan a get-together, or invite them to an event. It might mean addressing some emotional elephant in the room like a recent argument or a snarky comment. (That could require some additional preparation, and we'll talk about navigating disagreements and emotional challenges like this in coming chapters.)

There are some nuts and bolts to this kind of effort. You have to actually make that call, take out your calendar, clear that evening, and make plans. Preferably recurring plans!

But even with your most positive relationships, some of the old habits, the old automatic ways of being and interacting that make the relationship less energizing, may resurface. What follows are a few broad principles that we've found both in research and therapy to be effective in enlivening and energizing relationships:

Suggestion #1: The Power of Generosity

In the Western world, with its emphasis on individualism, the myth of the "self-made" man or woman gets a lot of airtime. Many of us imagine that our identity is self-created, that we are who we are because we made ourselves that way. In reality, we are who we are because of where we stand in relation to the world and to other people. The spoke of a wheel, if not attached to a wheel, is just a piece of metal. Even a hermit living in a cave is defined by his relation to, and distance from, other people.

Relationships are necessarily reciprocal systems. Support goes both ways. The support we receive is rarely an exact mirror image of the support we provide, but the old adage "you get what you give" is a good general rule.

This idea of giving what you'd like to receive in return is one answer to the powerlessness and hopelessness that people sometimes feel when they think of their relationships. We can't directly control the way other people engage with us, but we can control the way we engage with them. We may not be receiving a certain kind of support, but that doesn't mean we can't give it.

The Dalai Lama reminds us that what goes around comes around. "We are self-centered and selfish, but we need to be wisely selfish, not foolishly so," he once said. "If we neglect others, we too lose. . . . We can educate people to understand that the best way to fulfill their own interest is to be concerned about the welfare of others. But this will take time."

Research clearly shows that he's right: helping others benefits the one who helps. There is both a neural and a practical link between generosity and happiness. Being generous is a way to prime your brain for good feelings, and those good feelings in turn make us more likely to help others in the future. Generosity is an upward spiral.

Go back through the questions about support from earlier in the chapter and, thinking honestly about yourself, answer them in the opposite direction: Do you provide these types of support to others? If so, to whom? Are there people in your life you want to support more? Recall Kiecolt-Glaser's research on caregiver stress and wound healing from earlier in this chapter. If you have people in your life who are caring for others, or who are under major life stress, are there ways you can be there for them, and make sure they are receiving support themselves? If you are a caregiver, are you getting the support you need? As you look over your social universe, how does the balance of giving and receiving feel?

PEOPLE I SUPPORT

My Relationship With	Safety and Security	Learning and Growth	Emotional Closeness and Confiding	Identity Affirmation and Shared Experience	Romantic Intimacy	Help (Both Info and Practical)	Fun and Relaxation

Suggestion #2: Learning New Dance Steps

We get better at what we practice, and without realizing it we can become very talented at doing things that are not in our interest. Sterling Ainsley, for example, had gotten better and better at avoiding closeness and connection. He had good reason; even though he had his sister, Rosalie, there with him during the first years of his life, she couldn't stop his father's abuse, and his family of origin was pulled apart when his father committed his mother to the sanitarium. When Sterling moved to the farm, he could no longer see Rosalie on a regular basis, and this was painful to him. So he carried his fears of close relationships far into his adult life. With the exception of his adoptive mother, he never established that crucial sense of safety and security with another person, let alone with multiple people. Without necessarily articulating it to himself, he lived his life assuming that he would be happier, or at least safer, without close contacts. Being close to others, he believed, was a risk.

He was right, in a way. Our strongest feelings emerge from our connections with other people, and while the social world is filled with pleasures and meaning, it also contains doses of disappointment and pain. We get hurt by the people we love. We feel the sting when they disappoint us or leave us, and the emptiness when they die.

The impulse to avoid these negative experiences in relationships makes sense. But if we want the benefits of being involved with other people, we have to tolerate a certain amount of risk. We also have to be willing to see beyond our own concerns, and our own fears.

This raises that important question of how someone with Sterling's traumatic history can keep from letting it dominate their life. We hope he would have good experiences of closeness as he got older that would change his reigning paradigm. It happens. A positive, trusting relationship with a spouse can make a less secure person feel more secure. But too many people with Sterling's history just move from one self-fulfilling prophecy to another and never have a different experience of closeness.

The question is, how do we keep from always fighting the last traumatic battle and open ourselves to new experience?

Suggestion #3: Radical Curiosity

> Every man I meet is my master in some point, and in that I learn of
> him.
>
> Ralph Waldo Emerson

We often struggle in relationships for the same reason we struggle in other areas of life: we become too self-focused. We worry about whether we're doing it right, whether we're good at something, whether we're getting what we want. Like Sterling, or John Marsden, the unhappy lawyer, when we become too self-focused, we can forget about the experiences of others.

It's a common trap, but it's not inevitable. The same curiosity that makes us want to experience something new in a book or a movie can inform how we approach our relationships in even the most routine moments of life.

It can be a real joy to lose ourselves in the experience of another person. It can also feel strange at first, if you're not used to it, and it might take some effort. *Curiosity—real, deep curiosity about what others are experiencing— goes a long way in important relationships.* It opens up avenues of conversation and knowledge that we never knew were there. It helps others feel understood and appreciated. It's important even in less significant relationships, where it can set a precedent of caring and increase the strength of new, fragile bonds.

Maybe you know someone in your life who is always talking to people, rooting out their stories and opinions. It's no coincidence that these people are often very joyful and alive. Just as the "strangers on a train" experiment we mentioned in Chapter Two demonstrated, interacting with other people improves our mood and makes us happier than we expect it will.

Bob thinks of his father, who would talk to strangers everywhere. He was obsessively—radically—curious about everyone. Bob's aunt and uncle often told a story about how they once got into a cab with him in Washington, D.C. Bob's father sat in the front, as always, so he could talk to the driver. While he was extracting this man's entire life story, he started play-ing with the quarter-glass window that used to be a feature in old cars. He was so absorbed in the conversation that he didn't realize the window had come off in his hand. Peals of laughter were coming from the backseat, but Bob's father was too absorbed in his conversation to notice. He set the little window on the seat beside him and started playing with the window crank, which also came off. He set that down, too, and just kept asking questions. Lucky for the car it was a short drive.

This behavior came naturally to him. He didn't necessarily do it to be kind to people, he did it because it made him feel good. It energized him. Some of us are out of practice and have forgotten how this kind of curios-ity can feel, so we have to be more deliberate. We have to take an almost radical approach to cultivating the often subtle seeds of our natural inter-est in people, and take a bold step beyond our usual conversation habits. We need to make a point to ask ourselves: Who is this person, really, and what's their deal? Then it's as simple as asking a question, listening to the reply, and seeing where it takes us.

The crucial point is that being curious helps us connect to others, and this connection makes us more engaged with life. Genuine curiosity in-vites people to share more of themselves with us, and this in turn helps us understand them. This process enlivens everyone involved. The "strang-ers on a train" experiment points to these cascading benefits, which we'll discuss much more in Chapter Ten. Even a small interest in another per-son, a brief word, can create new excitements, new avenues of connection, and new pathways for life to flow.

Like generosity, curiosity is an upward spiral.

FROM CURIOSITY TO UNDERSTANDING

When people hear that we, Bob and Marc, are therapists, they often react by saying something like, "How can you listen to other people's problems all the time? That must be exhausting and depressing." It's true that listen-ing isn't always easy, but the more prevalent and powerful experience for both of us is one of gratitude to the people we work with in therapy. We learn from their experience and it deepens our connection to them. One of our greatest joys (and this is not confined to therapy) comes in moments when we sense that we've understood the experience of another person and then communicated that understanding in a way that feels true to them. It's life-affirming to suddenly find oneself in sync with the experience of someone else.

This is a crucial step in connecting with others through curiosity: communicating your new understanding back to them. This is where a lot of the magic happens, where the connection between people becomes solid, visible, and meaningful. Hearing an accurate understanding of our own experience coming from another person, articulated in their words, can be thrilling, especially when we're feeling alienated in a social setting. Suddenly someone is seeing us as we are, and that experience momentarily breaches the barrier that we feel between us and the world. To be seen is an amazing thing.

Conversely, it's an amazing thing to really see another person, and to communicate that new sight. The thrill of connection happens both for the person being seen and the person doing the seeing. Again, the connection and the feeling of vitality go both ways.

This is not a new or unconventional idea. The classic and hugely influential Dale Carnegie book *How to Win Friends and Influence People*, written in 1936, emphasized this point. The book is based on six principles, and the very first is "Become genuinely interested in other people." As with anything, the more you practice this kind of curiosity, the easier it gets. And the materials for practice are almost always available. You can make a choice right now, today, even in the next few minutes, that will move you in the right direction.

TAKING IT BACK TO LIFE

Just as maintaining social fitness requires some regular exercise, reflecting on all of your relationships benefits from regular check-ins. Don't hesitate to do it again in the future. If your social fitness is not where you would like it to be, you might want to do these reflective check-ins even more often. It never hurts—especially if you've been feeling low—to take a minute to reflect on how your relationships are faring and what you wish could be different about them. If you're the scheduling type, you could make it a regular thing; perhaps every year on New Year's Day or the morning of your birthday, take a few moments to draw up your current social universe, and consider what you're receiving, what you're giving, and where you would like to be in another year. You could keep your chart or relationships assessment somewhere private, or even right here in this book, so you know where to look the next time you want to peek at it to see how things have changed. A lot can happen in a year.

If nothing else, doing this reminds us of what's most important; always a good thing. Over and over again, when the participants in the Harvard Study reached their 70s and 80s, they would make a point to say that what they valued most were their relationships with friends and family. Sterling Ainsley himself made that point. He loved his adoptive mother and sister deeply—but he lost touch with them. Some of his fondest memories were of his friends—whom he never contacted. There was nothing he cared more about than his children—whom he rarely saw. From the outside it might look like he didn't care. That was not the case. Sterling was quite emotional in his recounting of his most cherished relationships, and his reluctance to answer certain Study questions was clearly connected to the pain that keeping his distance had caused him over the years. Sterling never sat down to really think about how he might conduct his relationships, or what he might do to properly care for the people he loved most.

If we accept the wisdom—and more recently the scientific evidence—that our relationships really are among our most valuable tools for sustaining health and happiness, then choosing to invest time and energy in them becomes vitally important. And an investment in our social fitness isn't only an investment in our lives as they are now. It is an investment that will affect everything about how we live in the future.

ATTENTION TO RELATIONSHIPS

Your Best Investment

The only gift is a portion of thyself.

Ralph Waldo Emerson

Harvard Study Second Generation Questionnaire, 2015

It seems I am "running on automatic" without much awareness of what I'm doing.

Never   Occasionally   Sometimes   Often   Always

I rush through activities without being really attentive to them.

Never   Occasionally   Sometimes   Often   Always

I pay attention to physical experiences, such as the wind in my hair or the sun on my face.

Never   Occasionally   Sometimes   Often   Always

Imagine you began your life with all the money you'll ever have. The instant you were born you were given one account, and anytime you've had to pay for something, it's come out of that account.

You don't need to work, but everything you do costs money. Food, water, housing, and consumer goods are as expensive as ever, but now even sending an email requires some of your precious funds. Sitting quietly in a chair doing nothing costs money. Sleep costs money. Everything you encounter requires you to spend money.

But the problem is this: you don't know how much money is in the account, and when it runs dry, your life is over.

If you found yourself in this circumstance, would you live in the same way? Would you do anything differently?

This is a fantasy, but change one key element and it's not far from our actual situation as human beings. Only instead of money, our one account has a limited amount of *time*—and we don't know how much.

It is an everyday sort of question—*How should we spend our time?*—but because of the brevity and uncertainty of life, it is also a profound question, and has major implications for our health and happiness.

There is a Buddhist mantra that monks are taught to use in meditation. It goes like this: "If only death is certain, and the time of death is uncertain, then what should I do?"

When you are confronted with an unavoidable awareness of the end of your own life, it imbues the world with a new perspective, and different things become important.

When we conducted our eight-day survey of Harvard Study couples in their 80s, at the end of each daily interview we asked them a different question about their perspectives on the life they'd lived so far. The value of time was often central to their answers:

DAY 7: As you look back on your life, what do you wish you had done less of? Had done more of?

> Edith, age 80: Less getting upset about silly things. When you put them into perspective, they weren't all that important. Less worrying about those things. More time with my children, husband, mother, father.
>
> Neil, age 83: Wish I'd spent more time with my wife. She died just as I'd begun to taper down with work.

These are only two of many similar responses. Nearly all Study participants were concerned about how they'd spent their time, and many felt that they hadn't given enough thought to what they paid attention to. It's an extremely common feeling. The flow of days has a way of whisking us away, so that we feel life is merely happening to us, that we are subjected to it, instead of actively shaping it. Like many people, some of our Study participants reached the late stages of their lives and looked back and had thoughts like, *I didn't see my friends enough . . . I didn't pay enough attention to my kids . . . So much of my time was spent doing things that weren't important to me.*

Note those verbs that we can't escape: We "spend" time, we "pay" attention.

Language—and perhaps English in particular—is so saturated with economic jargon that these words seem natural, they seem to make sense, but our time and attention are much, much more precious than these words suggest. *Time and attention are not something we can replenish. They are what our life is. When we offer our time and attention, we are not merely spending and paying. We are giving our lives.*

As the philosopher Simone Weil once wrote, "Attention is the rarest and purest form of generosity."

That's because attention—time—is the most valuable thing we possess.

Many decades after Simone Weil, the Zen master John Tarrant gave her insight a new dimension in his book *The Light Inside the Dark.* "Attention," he wrote, "is the most basic form of love."

We are pointing here to a truth that is difficult to put into words; like love, attention is a gift that flows both ways. When we give our attention, we are giving life, but we are also feeling more alive in the process.

Time and attention are the essential materials of happiness. They are the reservoir from which our lives flow. This is more accurate than any financial metaphor. Just as the water from a reservoir can be directed to, and enrich, particular areas of a landscape, the flow of our attention can enliven and enrich particular areas of our lives. So it never hurts to take a look at where our attention has been flowing, and ask if it's going into places that benefit both the people we love and ourselves (these two things usually go together). Are we thriving? Are the activities and pursuits that make us feel most alive getting their due share? Who are the people most important to us, and are those relationships, challenges and all, getting the attention they deserve?

NO TIME TODAY BUT PLENTY OF TIME TOMORROW

We are using the word "attention" in two different ways.

The first meaning of the word is really that of *priority* and *time spent.* This relates to the *frequency* dimension of the social universe chart from Chapter Four. Are we prioritizing the things that are most important to us, moving them to the front of the list when we apportion our time?

That's easy to say, you might be thinking, *but you obviously haven't seen my life. I can't just magically put more hours into the day. I'm investing my time in work so that my loved ones can eat and my kids have clothes to wear to school. I'm already stretched to the maximum, so how can I devote time that I don't have?*

It's a good question. So let's talk for a moment about time.

We often have two contradictory feelings about the time we have available to us. On one hand we sense a *time famine* and feel that there's just not enough time in the day to do everything that we need to do, let alone that we *want* to do. On the other hand, we tend to think that in some unspecified future we will have a *time surplus,* as if we'll get to a place in our lives where the kinds of things capturing our time right now will cease to consume us. That overdue visit to parents, that call to an old friend—anything we tend to imagine happening later—often gets the same treatment. "There'll be plenty of time later," we think, "for that."

It's true that large numbers of people report feeling too busy and overwhelmed with responsibilities and obligations. As the twenty-first century steamrolls ahead, it feels as if we have less and less time available, and those of us who feel time-poor are more stressed and less healthy. The most time-poor people in every society must be working longer and longer hours, right?

Not exactly. Globally, average work hours have declined significantly since the middle of the last century. Americans on average are working 10 percent less than they did in 1950, and in some countries like the Netherlands and Germany, working hours have been reduced by as much as 40 percent.

These are averages, and there are some caveats about who is working more, who is working less. For example, working mothers have the least leisure time, people with more education tend to work more and have less leisure time, and those with less education tend to have the most leisure time. So the picture isn't simple. But the data are clear: even considering the caveats, people are less busy with work than in recent generations, and yet we still feel that our time is stretched to the max. Why?

The answer to this question may lie in the second meaning of the word "attention," which is about *how* we spend time, and specifically, about *what our mind is doing* at any given moment.

THINKING ABOUT WHAT IS NOT HAPPENING

The two of us, Bob and Marc, have lived several hundred miles from each other for more than two decades. In order to work on projects together we have had to meet up by phone or video call. We're old friends but we have to set strict appointments, otherwise we'd never make it happen. When the appointment finally comes, at least once a week, we both see it like a scheduled respite in a hectic workweek. We relax a little bit and let down our guard. And sometimes, after being so focused all day or all week, when we're finally talking with each other, our attention wanders.

You know the feeling. Life is crazy, and there are always a million things to do. When you sit down with a friend, or with your kids, and you have a moment, your comfort and confidence in the relationship means you don't really *need* to pay full attention. These are the people you know. You have a routine together, the interaction is familiar, and maybe there's nothing particularly novel going on, so your mind kind of floats away. And even when our lives aren't flooded with worries and to-dos, there's always the vast flow of information on the internet calling to us. One moment of downtime in our day, and out comes the phone.

Even as we were working on this chapter, literally discussing the act of paying attention, Marc began to sense a familiar silence on the phone. Bob had spaced out.

"Bob," he said.

"Yes?"

"I've lost you."

It happens to everybody. In a 2010 study, Matthew Killingsworth and Daniel Gilbert turned one of the modern culprits of distraction—the smartphone—against itself, and used it to conduct a massive study of how we spend our waking moments, both physically and mentally. First they designed an app that contacted participants on their smartphones at random times throughout the day and presented them with questions about what they were doing, thinking, and feeling, recording their answers. The database collected millions of samples from more than five thousand people of all ages in eighty-three countries and across eighty-six occupational categories. Their findings showed that close to half of our waking moments are spent thinking about something other than what we are doing. Close to half! As the authors of the study point out, this is not just an unfortunate mental quirk, but a distinctly human evolutionary adaptation.

Thinking about the past and the future lets us plan, anticipate, and make creative connections among different ideas and experiences. But the modern environment, with all of its stimulation, may hold our minds in this state of distraction far beyond the point of diminishing returns. Our minds are not anticipating and making creative connections so much as wandering in the weeds. And the study by Killingsworth and Gilbert clearly showed what we are all dimly aware of—that *a wandering mind is connected to unhappiness.*

"The ability to think about what is not happening," they wrote, "is a cognitive achievement that comes at an emotional cost."

THE OWL AND THE HUMMINGBIRD

This cognitive ability to remember the past and anticipate the future is one reason some of us feel so busy—not because of the number of tasks we have to complete in the day, but because of the sheer number of things competing for our attention. What is commonly called "distraction" is probably better understood as overstimulation.

Recent findings in neuroscience have shown that our conscious minds cannot do more than one thing at a time. It may feel like you are able to multitask and think about two (or more) things at once, but really your mind is switching between them. This is a costly process neurologically speaking. Switching from one task to another takes energy and a measurable amount of time. Then, when we switch back, it takes *another* period of time to really wrap our minds around the original object of attention. And it's not only about the time cost; it's about the quality of our attention. If we are always switching from one thing to another, then we are never able to truly focus and experience the pleasure and effectiveness of a focused mind. Instead we live in a state of constant recalibration, or what the writer Linda Stone perceptively calls "continuous partial attention."

Human awareness is not the speedy, nimble creature some of us believe it to be. Our brains have evolved to be more like owls than hummingbirds: we notice something, turn our attention to it, and focus in. It is in this state of intense, solitary focus that we are in possession of our most uniquely human and powerful mental faculties. When we focus on one thing, we are at our most thoughtful, creative, and productive.

But in the screen-heavy environment of the twenty-first century, our mind-owls, large and unwieldy, are treated like hummingbirds, and they end up flopping ineffectively from one thing to the next. Doing this day in and day out accommodates us to what is actually an unnatural, anxiety-producing mode in which the mind struggles to find nourishment.

Which owl is going to feel busier, the one focusing on the sound of a mouse in the snow, or the one trying to draw tiny bits of nectar from a thousand flowers? And which owl is going to be, in the end, better nourished?

ONE FAMILY'S LIFE OF ATTENTION

Knowing that your attention is valuable is one thing, but what does attention look like in our relationships over the course of a lifetime?

For some real-world context, let's take a look at Leo DeMarco, our high school teacher from Chapter Two, who was generally considered to be one of the Harvard Study's happiest men, and how he managed his time and attention.

Leo was incredibly busy as a high school teacher and his time was stretched to the maximum. He was deeply involved with his students. More involved than most teachers, according to those who knew him. He always felt there was more to do, and never hesitated to help a student who was having a hard time or to meet with a concerned parent. He was also involved in extracurricular activities and so was not always available to his own children after school or on the weekends. His family enjoyed his company—he was a good listener, and always ready with a well-timed joke—so they noticed when he wasn't around and sometimes wondered if he valued his work more than his family.

It's true that his work was important to him. It gave his life meaning, and he told the Study more than once that it made him feel like a valuable member of the community, like he meant something to the people he worked with and especially to his students. This kind of purpose is important to our happiness and well-being (more on that in Chapter Nine), and it's not uncommon that it comes into conflict with other priorities, like family time. This competition for our attention is a tricky challenge that a lot of us find ourselves grappling with. But it's not insurmountable.

Leo's family was not afraid to share their feelings about this. His wife, Grace, mentioned it to him, and his two daughters and son mentioned it also.

In 1986 his oldest daughter, Katherine, was asked about the strongest memories she had of Leo, and she talked with great feeling about their fishing trips. Every summer, when he was not teaching, Leo would take one child at a time for a week to different camping spots and fishing holes. During these trips she remembered him being attentive to her, not just fishing, and asking about her life and what she thought of things. Unable to turn off the teacher in himself, he showed them how to tie on the hooks and bobbers, where the fish liked to hide out, how to build a fire, and how to identify constellations in the night sky. He made sure they would all be able to camp and fish on their own, so they could handle themselves in the wilderness and continue the tradition with their own kids, should they ever have them.

Leo gave his children his focused attention, and he offered it to his wife, Grace, as well. In his early 80s, when Leo was asked what kinds of activities they did together as a couple, he said:

> We'll garden together or I'll just walk along with her and we just talk about the landscape. I mean, yesterday we went for a three- or four-mile hike. Bundled up, deep in the woods, and we kept stopping and watching the ducks fly out of the creek that we were crossing over. There's a lot of that in my life. These are things that we share. Or when I read a book, I know what kinds of things appeal to her so I can suggest that she take a look at something. And she does the same for me.

These are small things, small moments in the days of Leo and Grace's life, but taken together over a lifetime, these small moments add up. "Attention is the most basic form of love." It's not a coincidence that Leo is both one of the more attentive, present members of the Study and one of its happiest.

THE MODERN MEANS OF CONNECTION

To Leo and other First Generation Harvard Study participants who were raising their kids in the 1940s, 1950s, and 1960s, the online life we know in the twenty-first century would have sounded like science fiction. Back then, they didn't have to contend with the omnipresence of smartphones, the pervasive nature of social media, or the overwhelming glut of information and stimuli. But their struggles with relationships might have more in common with the struggles of today than it first appears.

In 1946, a young Stanley Kubrick published a photo in *Look* magazine that would be very familiar today: a subway car full of New York City commuters, heads bowed, nearly every single one of them absorbed in . . . their newspapers. And many original Harvard Study families talked about having the same feelings many of us have today—they struggled to give their families the attention they deserved, work was overwhelming, the world seemed to be going crazy, and they were worried for their children's future. Remember, 89 percent of the Study's college men served in World War II—a catastrophic conflict the outcome of which, at the time, was entirely uncertain—and then raised children amidst the Cold War and pervasive fears of nuclear disaster. Inside the home, instead of the internet, parents were worried about what television was doing to their kids, and to society in general. So while their challenges might have been different in nature and scale, and the speed of cultural change may have been, at least in some ways, less extreme than what we experience, the effective *solutions* for nourishing relationships—devoting time and attention in the present moment—were the same as they are today. Attention is the actual stuff of life, and it's equally valuable no matter what era a person lives in.

OUR ATTENTION, ONLINE

Technologies like the smartphone and social media now play a role in shaping some of the most intimate parts of our lives. Quite often, when we connect with another person, there is a device and a piece of software between us.

This is a vulnerable situation; an incredible amount of emotion and life flow through these media. The kindling of romance, breakups, news of births and deaths, the basic conduct of friendships, and all kinds of other intimate interactions are now filtered through devices and software whose design subtly—and sometimes not-so-subtly—shapes each interaction. How is this affecting our relationships? Our happiness? Are these new forms of communication *deepening* or *inhibiting* our ability to meaningfully connect to each other?

Definitive answers to these questions are not easy to come by. Every individual uses these technologies differently, and as with any period of social transformation, the true nature of change is hard to see until we have some distance to look back on it. But one thing we do know is that social media and online life are complicated. There are reasons to be hopeful, and reasons to worry.

THE GIVE-AND-TAKE OF SOCIAL MEDIA

On the positive side, when social media is used to sustain relationships with friends and family, it can enhance feelings of connectedness and belonging. Old friends and colleagues that we may have lost touch with in the past are now only a few clicks away, and new communities emerge every day around interests and challenges. Someone with a rare disease like cystic fibrosis can find support and comfort online, and someone who has been marginalized because of their sexual orientation, gender identity, or the way they look can find a community beyond their physical location. For anyone who is isolated and in an unusual situation, the internet is a true blessing.

But there are important questions to ask, and the answers may have implications for our personal well-being and for society. Among the most urgent is how these online spaces affect the way children and adolescents develop. As data from our own Harvard Study (and many others) have shown, early social experiences matter. A person's style of relating to others later in their life is linked to how they developed as children. We call them *the formative years* for a reason (more on this in Chapter Eight). What impact does more online interaction have on young people's ability to read social cues and recognize emotions in real life? Or on their ability to give meaningful conversational cues and emotional signals? A great deal of in-person communication has nothing to do with language. Do these nonverbal abilities atrophy in virtual contexts in ways that affect in-person interactions?

This is a rich and developing area of research, some of which we are conducting ourselves. The results so far are not conclusive; much more research must be done. But what's clear at this point is that we can't assume that online spaces are the same as physical spaces, and we especially can't assume that the social skills kids develop by being together in person are skills they can also develop online.

ISOLATION AND CONNECTION

In 2020 the world was rocked by the Covid-19 pandemic. The rapid spread of a microscopic virus drastically changed much of the world's way of life, separating us from our friends, neighbors, and families, and taxing our individual psychological fortitude to the extreme. Quarantines drove people into their homes, and social distancing rules prevented most forms of socializing. Restaurants shut down. Workplaces closed. Almost overnight, online video calls and social media became many people's only connection to the outside world. It was like a massive global experiment in both social isolation and the nature of life online.

As weeks of lockdown stretched into months, online tools began to fill the void left by a lack of real-world interaction. Remote meetings kept many businesses afloat and allowed schools and universities to keep their (virtual) doors open. Religious services were held online. Even weddings and funerals were conducted virtually.

But for those who lacked internet access, the situation was more dire. Faced with total isolation or the risk of infection, many people chose to risk infection. In nursing homes where social media and video calling were rare, the only thing worse than the virus was the social isolation, which was so damaging to residents' health that it became an official cause of death.

Without social media and video calling, it's likely that the health effects of the lockdown would have been much more severe.

But it soon became clear that these virtual tools were far from sufficient. Something was missing in the feeling of these online meetings, in their sensory experience and emotional content.

Communication is not only an exchange of information. Human touch and physical proximity have emotional, psychological, and even biological effects. Boxed in by the capabilities of software, the experience of social interaction online is different and often more constrained. Whereas in normal times the limitations of online connection are offset by regular in-person interactions, during the pandemic these limitations were placed into stark relief. Despite our virtual connectedness, diseases of despair, depression, and anxiety increased in the first year of pandemic, and feelings of loneliness worsened in some communities. Even among those most well-connected online, many began to experience "skin hunger," a longing driven by the deprivation of human touch. In the face of intense isolation, social media was at least *something*. But it wasn't enough.

This massive global experiment in isolation made one thing very clear: the physical presence of another human being cannot be duplicated by a machine. There is no substitute for being together.

DON'T SCROLL, ENGAGE

Social media and virtual interaction are here to stay, and they are likely to evolve in unpredictable ways. As we watch the way societies all over the world cope with these technological changes, is there anything we can do in our own lives to magnify the good and mitigate the bad?

Thankfully, we do have some data on this. How an individual uses these platforms matters, and we have a couple of very basic recommendations that you can implement today:

First, *engage with others.*

One influential study showed that those who use Facebook passively, just reading and scrolling, feel worse than those who engage actively by contacting others and commenting on posts. A similar conclusion was reached in a study in Norway, one of the "happiest" countries on the planet. Norwegians use Facebook at high rates, children especially, and one study found that the kids who used Facebook primarily to communicate experienced more positive feelings. The kids who used it primarily to observe experienced more negative feelings. These findings are not that surprising: we now know that those who compare themselves to others more frequently are less happy.

As we said earlier, we are always comparing our insides to other people's outsides, always comparing our own experiences of ups and downs, good days and bad days, feelings of confidence and insecurity, with the curated version of life that others show us. This happens most starkly on social media, where we're quick to post photos of a good time at a restaurant or beach vacation, but rarely balance those out with the reality of dinner table arguments or bad hangovers. This imbalance means that when we compare our lives with the pictures that others show us on social media, it's easy to feel like the good life is something that only other people are enjoying.

Second, *take your temperature when using social media.*

When it comes to social media, one size does not fit all. What's good for someone else may not be good for you. So when you're thinking about your own habits online, how you *feel* really matters. When you spend half an hour on Facebook, do you come away feeling energized? Do you feel depleted after a long click-hole journey around the internet? Taking a moment to notice the changes in your mood and outlook after a period of time on Facebook or Twitter can point you in the right direction. Next time you find yourself pinned to your chair by a screen, just take a second and check in with yourself; how do you feel?

Third, *check in with how your social media use is seen by people who are important to you.* Ask your partner how they feel about the way you use your phone. Are your online habits affecting them? Are there certain times or certain activities—at breakfast, after dinner, in the car—during which they miss your full attention and presence? What about your kids? Older people tend to assume that it's primarily kids that are glued to screens, but it's not uncommon at all for kids to complain about their parents' obsession with their smartphones. This isn't something that you can always perceive yourself; you might need to ask.

Finally, *take tech holidays.* These will vary depending on your life, but making a point to clear technology out of your life for small periods of time can reveal how it is affecting you. In science, we use a control group to stand in relief against the treatment group so any effect can be clearly seen. In your life, you might need a control period. What does it feel like to refrain from looking at social media for four hours? If your phone is unavailable, are you more attentive to the people you love? After a day free of social media, do you feel less overwhelmed, less scattered?

Anytime we pick up a smartphone or go online, we are increasing our potential reach and opening ourselves to vulnerabilities. The best that each of us can do is to try to understand how both sides of this equation map onto our own lives, and strive to maximize the good and mitigate the bad.

To that end, we have one crucial advantage over all of the tech giants: the war for our attention is being fought on our home turf; quite literally, in our minds. And it can be won there.

BEING (AND STAYING) ALERT

The present moment is the only time over which we have dominion.

Thich Nhat Hanh

These dilemmas of attention may seem unique to the modern moment, but at their core they are very old, millennia older than the internet, and they have very old solutions.

In 1979, Jon Kabat-Zinn adapted ancient Buddhist meditation practices into an eight-session course designed to help terminally ill patients and those with chronic pain reduce feelings of stress. He called the course "Mindfulness-Based Stress Reduction," or MBSR, and its therapeutic success led to the word "mindfulness" becoming the almost ubiquitous term it is today. A great deal of research now supports its effectiveness, and a large number of medical schools now offer mindfulness training.

At its core the practice of mindfulness is about alertness and attention. Kabat-Zinn often defines mindfulness in this way: "the awareness that emerges through paying attention on purpose, in the present moment, and non-judgmentally to things as they are." By making a conscious effort to pay attention to the sensations of our bodies and what is happening around us, and doing it without the abstraction and filter of judgment, our thinking and experience are brought into sync with where we are right now. The human mind has a tendency to run away; the goal of mindfulness is to keep bringing it back home, to the present moment.

Over the years, elements of mindfulness have permeated the broader culture, and efforts to commercialize it have led some to distrust mindfulness practices. But its core concepts have been around for centuries and are part of many cultural traditions. The goal is simply an everyday sort of attentiveness. Even the U.S. military is invested in mindfulness and learning how to keep human beings focused, because being alert to the moment, for a soldier, is a matter of life and death.

The same can be said for the rest of us. Being alert is the feeling of actually living. Accumulated moments of autopilot (for example, a mindless daily commute plus hours of surfing the internet plus the automatic routines around waking and going to sleep) contribute to the feeling that life is racing by and that we're missing it as it happens.

By learning to pay attention to what's happening in front of us, we gain more than the sensations of life; we also increase our ability to act. We're not thinking about what's already happened, about what might happen, about what we have to do later; we are alert to the moment, which is where any action must take place. If our intention is to connect with other people, being present is what makes that possible.

A moment of mindfulness needn't be a strenuous act of meditation. We need only to stop, pay attention, and notice things as they are. An amazing amount of information is available in every fleeting moment of our lives. You can take a moment right now, in the place you are. You can notice the weight of this book in your hand, the feel of the page (or of the device you are using to read or listen to it), the movement of the air across your skin, or the play of light on the floor of the room. Or you can try asking yourself this lovely question, which is useful in any situation, at any time: *What's here that I've never noticed before?*

The word "mindfulness" is unfortunate in a way, because its meaning may not be evident to some people. The word seems to suggest that the practice is about thinking the right things, that if we are mindful it means our mind is "full" of the right thoughts.

But mindfulness is simpler than that.

As the Gilbert and Killingsworth study showed, more often than not, most people's minds are already full of thought—about ourselves, the future, and the past. This kind of thinking pulls our minds into a narrow tunnel made of thought and worry, cut off from immediate experience. It can be dark and claustrophobic there.

The present moment is large and spacious, if we allow it to be. Even when it contains sad or scary experiences, this moment includes so much more than the content of our minds. The sense of being truly alive comes with giving our attention only to what is happening right in front of us, to grab hold of sensations—the feelings of our bodies, the things we see and hear, the presence of the people who are with us—and use them to make a hard left out of thinking about other things and places, and to emerge from the tunnel of our own minds into the vastness of the present, the only place anything, or anyone, really exists.

As the spiritualist Ram Dass simply put it, the idea is to "be here now."

"A" FOR EFFORT

That same question—What's here that I'm not noticing?—can be extraordinarily powerful when we apply it to people: What about this person have I not noticed before? Or: What is this person feeling that I've been missing? This is part of that radical curiosity we talked about in Chapter Four.

More often than not, when we are in the presence of other people, we are missing *a lot* about their experience. In any interaction, and in any relationship (even our closest), there is an enormous amount of feeling and information that goes right over our heads. But in the end, which matters more: How right we are about what another person is experiencing, or how curious we are about their experience in the first place?

In 2012 the two of us designed a study to help work this out. If you've ever had a difficult conversation with a romantic partner, you know how fraught that can be, and how much misunderstanding can go on. So we recruited 156 couples from diverse backgrounds, and asked each partner to record a one- or two-sentence summary about a relationship event in the past month that frustrated, angered, or disappointed them (for example, the partner did not follow through on something they had promised, did not share information about an important event, did not do a household task that was theirs to do). Then we played each partner's recording for the couple to initiate a discussion, and we instructed them to try to come to a better understanding of what occurred.

The participants didn't know this, but we were tracking the importance of empathy. What we wanted to know was this: Is it more important to be *accurate* in our understanding of our partner's feelings, or is it more important that our partners see that we are making an *effort to understand*?

After their interaction, we asked them about both their own and their partner's feelings during these conversations. We also asked a series of questions about their partner's intentions and motivations, including the degree to which they felt their partner was trying to understand them.

We expected that *empathic accuracy*—getting the right answer about what your partner was feeling—would correlate with a stronger sense of relationship satisfaction. This correlation was certainly there— understanding how your partner is feeling is a good thing.

But more important than that, especially for women, was the *empathic effort* involved. If a person felt their partner was making a good-faith effort to understand them, they felt more positively about the interaction and about the relationship, regardless of their partner's accuracy.

To put it simply, understanding another person is great, but just *trying to understand* goes a long way in building connection.

Some people do this automatically, but efforts to understand others can also be deliberate, intentional behaviors. It needn't come naturally to you at first, but the more you try, the easier it will get. The next time you have the opportunity, try asking yourself:

How is this person feeling?
What is this person thinking?
Am I missing something here?
How might I feel if I were in this person's shoes?

And when you can, let them know that you're curious and trying to understand—a small effort that can have an enormous impact.

LEO GETS A B+ FOR EFFORT

Leo may not have been the Study member who spent the *most time* with his family, but over the years he made a conscious attempt to improve in that area, and when he did spend time with them, he made it count. That doesn't mean that he took them on spectacular adventures or international trips, or that he crammed the maximum amount of excitement into every moment of family time. No. He paid attention to his children and his wife and he did so relatively consistently. He was available to them, in the moment. He listened, he asked questions, and he made a point to help whenever he could.

We asked him what had appealed to him about his wife when they first met in high school, and he listed a number of things: her intelligence, her ease of manner, and something mysterious that he couldn't put his finger on—"just something that I liked about her. I liked her right from the start." But when we asked him what he thought *she* liked about *him*, the question startled him.

"Well I've never thought about that, to be honest," he said. He was so interested in Grace that he hadn't thought about how he appeared to her.

This focus on the world outside of himself is a theme in Leo's life. When his family all got together, he said he enjoyed being a fly on the wall. Their relationships with each other were fun for him to watch, to see them in their natural states, how they were different with each other than with him. Their relationships infused the household with energy. "It makes life wonderful," he said.

Leo was lucky. His curiosity, attention to others, and lack of self-consciousness were natural for him. These do not come as naturally to everyone. Some of us have to make a more deliberate effort and learn to be attentive in this way. Even Leo, who remained attentive to his wife throughout his life, didn't keep up his proactive approach to connecting with his children. He talked with them less and less after they left home, and in general was less attentive. When she was in her mid-30s, his youngest daughter, Rachel, wrote an unprompted note on her Second Generation questionnaire:

> Adore both parents. Just realized this year that I have to carve time out to be with them, especially to get my father to talk. He has always let my mother do the necessary communicating. Now I initiate great late-night conversations, and feel much closer to him.

This comment is very revealing. The DeMarco family was close to each other, it's true, but sometimes that's not enough. After Rachel became an adult, she lost some of that closeness with her parents in a way that didn't feel good to her. She had to become more active in making time for them, and in nurturing her relationship with her father. As a family, they already had the ability to communicate and to be close, and yet effort and planning were still necessary. Closeness didn't just happen on its own. Life is busy. So many things get in the way, and it's easy to become passive and just go with the flow. Rachel made a choice to move against the flow of her life and reconnect.

Rachel's choice didn't come out of nowhere. Leo may not have known it when he was a young father, but he was sowing the seeds of connection that would come back and nourish him (and his kids) later in life. Rachel and his other children learned that this kind of connection with their father felt good and gave their lives a special feeling they couldn't easily get from anyone else. They knew this because of Leo's earlier efforts.

At the very end of her questionnaire, Rachel made a final note to Study researchers:

> p.s. Sorry this is late, I live in the deep woods on a mountain, no H2O, electricity, etc. A bit cut-off!

. . . so it seems more than one lesson from their camping trips took hold.

A close look at the DeMarco family reveals what research also shows are some of the natural outgrowths of focused attention: reciprocal love and consideration, a sense of belonging, and positive feeling about human relationships in general—which then leads to more positive relationships, and better health. In the case of Leo and the DeMarco family, their close attention to each other seems to have had a major impact on all of their lives.

A LITTLE MORE ATTENTION, EVERY DAY

We've already asked you to consider the relationships in your life that could use some more time. Now we're going to ask you to consider a deeper question: Of the people in your life who are already receiving your time, who among them is receiving your full *attention*?

This question may be more difficult to answer than you think. We often believe that we are giving our full attention, but our automatic actions and reactions make it hard to know for sure. You might have to make an effort to observe yourself and to consider if you really are offering the people who are most important to you the fullness of your attention.

How you do this will be particular to your own life, but here are a few simple ways to begin.

First, think of one or two relationships that enrich your life, and consider devoting some extra attention to them. If you made a social universe chart in Chapter Four, you might take a look at it and ask yourself, *What action could I take today to give attention and appreciation to someone who deserves it?*

Second, consider some changes to your day. Is it practical to create some time or activities that are distraction-free, particularly when you are with the people you care most about? For example, no phones at the dinner table? Are there set times in the week or in the month that you can dedicate to a certain person? Can a change in your daily schedule lead to a regular time for coffee or a walk with a loved one or a new friend? Can you arrange a few pieces of furniture to facilitate conversation rather than facilitate screen time?

Finally, you might continue the practice we began in Chapter Four, and bring some curiosity to each moment you have with the people in your life, especially those you know well and perhaps take for granted. This takes practice, but it's not hard to get better at it. *"How was your day?"*— *"Fine"* needn't be the end of a conversation. It is your sincere interest that will motivate folks to respond. You might follow up with something a little more playful like, *"What was the most fun thing that happened today?"*

Or, *"Did anything surprising happen today?"* And when someone makes a casual reply you can dig deeper: *"Can I ask you more about that . . . I'm so curious and not sure I really understand it fully . . ."* Try to put yourself in this person's place and imagine what they have experienced. Engaging conversations often come from this perspective-taking alone, and curiosity can be contagious. You might find that the more interested you are in others, the more interested they become in you, and you might also be surprised how fun this process can be.

Life is always at risk of slipping by unnoticed. If the days and months and years feel as if they are moving too quickly, focused attention might be one remedy. Giving something your undivided attention is a way of bringing it to life and assuring that you don't float through time on automatic pilot. Noticing someone is a way of respecting them, paying tribute to the person they are in that exact moment. And noticing yourself, checking in about how you move through the world, about where you are now and where you would like to be, can help you identify which people and pursuits most need your attention. Attention is your most precious asset, and deciding how to invest it is one of the most important decisions you can make. The good news is you can make that decision now, in this moment, and in each moment of your life.

FACING THE MUSIC

Adapting to Challenges in Your Relationships

There is a crack, a crack in everything
That's how the light gets in.

Leonard Cohen

Harvard Study Questionnaire, 1985, Section VI

Q#8: What is your philosophy for getting over the rough spots?

At age 26, Peggy Keane seemed to everyone who knew her to be well on the path to a good life. She had a promising career, and a loving family. We heard from her in Chapter Three as she told us about her marriage to a man she described as "one of the nicest men on the planet." But this picture of her life did not match the deeper reality. Only a few months after her wedding, Peggy's life fell into disarray when she acknowledged to herself, her husband, and her family that she was gay. Peggy had been hiding this truth about herself for years, and when she finally turned to face it, her entire world seemed to collapse. She felt alone, out of energy, and out of resources. It was the most difficult moment of her life. When she came up for air after that period of confusion and despair, she looked around at her life and thought, *What now? Who can I turn to?*

Throughout this book, we've been emphasizing that relationships are the key not only to navigating difficulties, big and small, but to flourishing in the face of them. George Vaillant summed this point up well when he wrote: "There are two pillars of happiness revealed by the [Harvard Study]. . . . One is love. The other is finding a way of coping with life that does not push love away."

It is within our relationships—and especially our close relationships—that we find the ingredients of the good life. But getting there isn't simple. When we look across the eighty-four years of the Harvard Study, we can see that the happiest and healthiest participants were those with the best relationships. But when we examine the lowest moments in our participants' lives, a great deal of them *also* involve relationships. Divorces, the death of loved ones, challenges with drugs and alcohol that pushed key relationships to the brink . . . many of the hardest times in participants' lives have been the result of their love for and closeness to other people.

It's one of the great ironies of life—and the subject of millions of songs, films, and great works of literature—that the people who make us feel the most alive and who know us best are also the people able to hurt us most. This doesn't mean that the people who hurt us are malicious, or that we are acting maliciously when we hurt others. Sometimes there is no fault. As we travel on our own unique paths, we can hurt each other without intending to.

This is the conundrum we find ourselves in as human beings, and how we deal with challenges often defines the course of our lives. Do we face the music? Or do we bury our heads in the sand?

What did Peggy do?

Let's fast-forward in Peggy's life to March of 2016, shortly after her 50th birthday, and take a look at how things worked out for her.

Throughout the 1990s, Peggy focused on her career. She completed a master's degree and started teaching. After one short relationship and a period of being single, Peggy fell in love in 2001 and has been in a close relationship with the same woman ever since. She describes her relationship as "very happy, warm, and comfortable." But in 2016 she'd been having some trouble at work, and the stress was affecting her life:

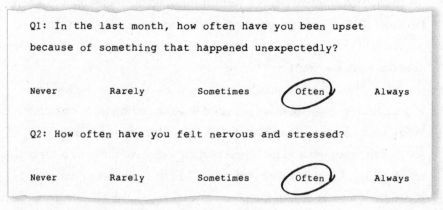

Q1: In the last month, how often have you been upset because of something that happened unexpectedly?

Never   Rarely   Sometimes   *Often*   Always

Q2: How often have you felt nervous and stressed?

Never   Rarely   Sometimes   *Often*   Always

But even though she'd been under pressure, Peggy wasn't particularly worried:

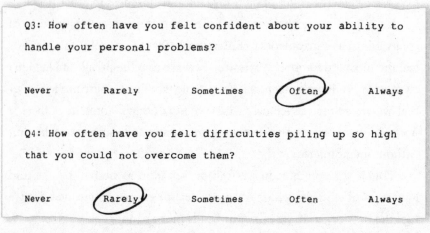

Q3: How often have you felt confident about your ability to handle your personal problems?

Never   Rarely   Sometimes   *Often*   Always

Q4: How often have you felt difficulties piling up so high that you could not overcome them?

Never   *Rarely*   Sometimes   Often   Always

What were the reasons for Peggy's confidence in tackling problems? In no small part, her friends and family:

Q.43: How much does each statement describe you?
Friends care about you.

Not at all A little bit   Some   Quite a bit   A lot

Family cares about you.

Not at all A little bit   Some   Quite a bit   A lot

Friends help you with serious problems.

Not at all A little bit   Some   Quite a bit   A lot

Family helps you with serious problems.

Not at all A little bit   Some   Quite a bit   A lot

Peggy went through the wringer and came out on the other side, and her relationships are what helped her through. Because of her full engagement with the people who are close to her, she's lived, as Zen Buddhists sometimes say, "the ten thousand joys and the ten thousand sorrows."

As we travel along our individual paths, one of the few things we can be absolutely sure of is that we will face challenges in life and in our relationships that we don't feel equipped to handle. The lives of two generations of Harvard Study participants broadcast this truth loudly and clearly. It doesn't matter how wise, how experienced, or how capable we are; we will sometimes feel overmatched. And yet if we are willing to face into these challenges, there is a tremendous amount that can be done. "You can't stop the waves," Jon Kabat-Zinn wrote, "but you can learn to surf."

In Chapter Five, we talked about the importance of paying attention to the present moment, and the incredible value of directing that attentiveness toward the people in our lives. Now the question becomes: What happens when we find ourselves in that present moment, engaged with people and experiencing significant challenges? Life happens only in the moment. If we're going to face the music, we have to do it one moment at a time, one interaction at a time, one feeling at a time.

This chapter is about these moment-to-moment choices and interactions, about living with and adapting to challenges in our relationships and in life, so that when the waves come crashing our way, rather than succumbing to them, we can meet them with all of the resources at our disposal, and ride.

REFLEXIVE VS. REFLECTIVE

Many difficulties in relationships stem from old habits. We develop automatic, reflexive behaviors over the course of our lives that become so intimately woven into our days that we don't even see them. In some cases, we become used to avoiding certain feelings and turning away, while in other cases we might be so overcome by emotion that we act on our feelings before we realize it.

The old phrase "knee-jerk reaction" is apt. When a doctor taps our knee in just the right spot, our nerves react and our foot kicks up. No thought or conscious effort is involved. Emotions often seem to affect us in the same way. A great deal of research has shown that once an emotion is elicited, our reactions are almost automatic. Emotional reactions are complex but include what researchers have called an "action tendency"— an urge to behave in a certain way. Fear, for example, includes an urge to escape. Emotions have evolved to enable rapid responses, particularly when we feel threatened. So when humans lived primarily in the wilderness, action tendencies had a strong survival benefit. Now things are less straightforward.

When Bob was a medical student, he encountered two cases that put into relief a crucial difference between more adaptive and less adaptive ways of coping with stress. Both involved women in their late 40s, each of whom had found a lump in her breast. We'll call them Abigail and Lucia. Abigail's initial reaction to the lump was to minimize its significance, and to tell no one. It was probably nothing, she decided. It was small, and whatever it was, it wasn't important. She didn't want to bother her husband or her two sons, who were away at college and busy with their own lives. After all, she felt fine and had other things to worry about.

Lucia's initial reaction was alarm. She told her husband, and after a brief conversation they agreed she should call her doctor and schedule an immediate appointment. Then she called her daughter and let her know what was going on. While she waited for the biopsy results to come back, she did her best to put it out of her mind so that she could get on with her life. She had a career, and other things to deal with. But her daughter called every day and her husband doted on her to the point that she had to ask him for some space.

Abigail and Lucia were both responding to an incredible stressor in ways that were natural for them. We all do this. Our habitual responses— patterns of both thinking and behaving—that arise when stressful events occur are what psychologists call *coping styles.*

Our coping styles affect the way we deal with every challenge that comes our way, from a minor disagreement to major catastrophe, and a key part of every coping style is how we use our relationships. Do we seek help? Do we accept help? Do we turn inward and face challenges in silence? Whatever coping style we use has an impact on those around us.

The coping styles of the two women that Bob encountered in his medical training could not have been more different. Abigail managed her fear by denying the significance of what she had discovered, and in this way she faced *away* from the difficulty. She did not involve her loved ones and did not take any action. She saw her situation as a potential burden on others. Lucia was also afraid, but she used her fear to face *toward* the difficulty and to take the actions necessary to preserve her health. She saw her situation as a matter that was larger than herself, something her family should face together. She *leaned in* to the situation, dealt with it directly, but remained flexible as well, managing the ebb and flow of the other demands of her life.

It turned out that both of these women had cancer. Abigail never told her family or her doctor what she had found and ignored the lump until she began to feel ill. By then it was too late, and the cancer took her life. Lucia caught the cancer early, went through a long course of treatment, and survived.

This is an extreme example, but this contrast in outcomes stuck with Bob for the clarity of its message: the inability or refusal to face challenges directly and to engage your support network can have enormous consequences.

FACING THE MUSIC VS. BURYING OUR HEADS IN THE SAND

Abigail's case is not unusual at all. Marc has helped run two separate studies designed to help women with breast cancer deal more directly with their fears and to access the support of important people in their lives. Among these women, Abigail's initial reaction—*avoidance*—was common.

It's often easier to turn away than it is to confront what troubles us. But doing so can have unintended consequences, and the effect of avoidance can be especially pronounced in the place it happens most: our personal relationships.

Many studies have shown that when we avoid confronting challenges in a relationship, not only does the problem not go away, but it can get worse. The original problem keeps burrowing down into the relationship and can lead to a variety of other problems.

This has been clear to psychologists for a long time, but what has been less clear is how this kind of avoidance can affect us over the course of life. Does a tendency to avoid dealing with challenges affect us only in the short term, or are there long-term consequences?

To get a lifetime perspective on this question, we used data from the

Harvard Study and asked, *What happens over the course of an entire life when a participant tends to face the music (lean in), and what happens when they tend to bury their heads in the sand (avoid)?* We found that a tendency to avoid thinking and talking about difficulties in middle age was associated with negative consequences more than thirty years later. Those people whose typical responses were to avoid or ignore difficulties had poorer memory and were less satisfied with their lives in late life than those who tended to face difficulties directly.

Of course, life is always bringing us new and different challenges. What served you well yesterday might not work today, and different kinds of relationships require different skills. The friendly joking to lighten an argument with your teenage child probably will not work with your neighbor who asks you to curb your dog. During a heated exchange at home, you might take your partner's hand; at work your boss might not appreciate the same gesture. We need to cultivate a variety of tools and use the right tool for the right challenge.

One lesson from research is that there are advantages to being flexible. There are men and women in the Harvard Study who are incredibly strong-willed. They have set ways of responding to challenges, and they stick to them. In some situations, they may find themselves in control, but in others they may be at a loss.

It was not uncommon in the 1960s, for example, for our First Generation Study participants to have difficulty finding common ground with their baby boomer children. This inability to adapt caused them stress.

"I don't like that hippy movement," Sterling Ainsley told the Study in 1967. "It disturbs me." He found himself alienated from his children, unable to be curious about their different views of the world.

Each of us has cultivated certain coping strategies through our lives, and they can become set in stone. This kind of "strength" can actually make us more fragile. In an earthquake, the sturdiest, most rigid structures are not the ones that survive. In fact, they might be the first to crumble. Structural science has figured this out, and building codes now require flexibility in tall structures, so that buildings are able to ride the literal wave rolling through the earth. The same with human beings. Being able to flex with changing circumstance is an incredibly powerful skill to learn. It might be the difference between getting through with minor damage and falling apart.

Changing our own automatic way of responding is not an easy thing to do. There are brilliant people in the Harvard Study—actual rocket scientists—who never managed even to recognize, much less control, their own coping strategies, and their lives were poorer for it. At the same time, participants like Peggy Keane, and her parents, Henry and Rosa, were able to grow by facing the trials of their lives as squarely as they could, and by using the support of friends and family.

So how do we move beyond our initial reactions when confronted by challenges?

When we are in the throes of emotional events, positive or negative, minor or major, our reactions often unfold so fast that we experience our emotions as if they are happening *to* us, and we are at their mercy. But in truth, our emotions are much more affected by our thinking than we realize.

There is now a great deal of research showing the connection between how we perceive events and how we feel about them. Humans understood this long before science developed the objective evidence.

"A happy heart is good medicine and a cheerful mind works healing," the Bible says, "but a broken spirit dries up the bones" (Proverbs 17:22).

The Stoic philosopher Epictetus noted that "Men are disturbed not by events, but by the views they take of them."

"Monks," the Buddha said, "we who look at the whole and not just the part, know that we too are systems of interdependence, of feelings, perceptions, thoughts, and consciousness all interconnected."

Our emotions need not be our masters; what we think, and how we approach each event in our lives, matters.

ONE MOMENT AT A TIME

If we take any emotional sequence—a *stressor* that evokes a *feeling* that elicits a *reaction* and its aftermath—and we zoom in and slow the sequence way down, a new hidden level of processing is revealed. Just as medical researchers find treatments for illness by looking at the smallest processes in the body, some surprising possibilities become available to us when we examine our emotional experience at a more microscopic level.

This process—from stressor to reaction—happens in stages. Each stage presents us with a range of choices that can propel us in a more positive or more negative direction, and each stage can be altered by our thinking or behavior.

Scientists have mapped these stages and used these maps to help children curb aggression, to help adults reduce depression, and to help athletes perform at peak efficiency. But these maps are useful for anyone in any emotional situation. By understanding how we move through these stages, and slowing them down, we can illuminate some of the mysteries behind why we feel the way we feel and do the things we do.

The model that follows provides a way for you to slow your reactions and put them under a microscope. We offer it as something you can keep in your back pocket (metaphorically) and use anytime, for any emotional situation. Our main focus in this book is on relationships, so we present examples of how this model can be used to respond to challenging experiences with other people. But it can be applied to challenges of all sorts—to unexpected and minor irritants like getting a flat tire, or to chronic health stressors like diabetes or arthritis. One moment at a time.

THE W.I.S.E.R. MODEL OF REACTING TO EMOTIONALLY CHALLENGING SITUATIONS AND RELATIONSHIP EVENTS

This model downshifts our typical reactions one or two gears and gives us a chance to look more closely at the rich particulars of situations, the experiences of other people, and our own reactions that we may have been missing.

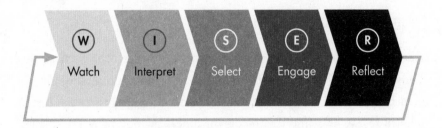

To show you how this model can be used in everyday life, we'll use a scenario we see a lot, both in our clinical practices and among participants in the Harvard Study: a family member who offers unwelcome advice.

Imagine a mother, we'll call her Clara, who has been having difficulty connecting with her teenage daughter, Angela. Angela is fifteen, and as most fifteen-year-olds do, she's striving to become more independent. She feels stifled by her mother and father and wants to spend time only with her friends. Angela has been a good student most of her life, but in the last year her grades have been slipping, she's been caught drinking several times, and she's been skipping classes, all of which have caused fights at home.

Angela's grandparents are sympathetic—Clara was defiant at that age herself—and they try to be supportive and leave the parenting to Clara. But Clara's older sister, Frances, also has teenage kids and thinks that Angela's parents are failing her. Aunt Frances worries about where Angela's headed and feels like it might be her duty to intervene.

At a family barbecue, Frances sees her niece Angela at the end of the picnic table, disengaged, texting with friends. "You know, smartphones kill the brain," she says, jokingly. "They've basically proved it in the lab." Then she says to her sister Clara, her tone still trying to communicate humor but with a hint of seriousness, "You wonder why her grades are slipping, maybe you should try disciplining her, take the phone away. That's what I do with my kids. Maybe then she'll have time for schoolwork."

Okay—so how could Clara use the W.I.S.E.R. model to help her decide how to respond to her sister?

Stage One: Watch (Curiosity Cures the Cat)

There's an old adage in psychiatry: Don't just do something, sit there.

Our initial impressions of a situation are powerful, but they are rarely complete. We tend to focus on the familiar, and this narrow view risks excluding potentially important information. Regardless of how much you can observe initially, there is almost always more to see. Whenever you encounter a stressor and you feel the emotion brewing, a bit of purposeful curiosity right away is useful. Thoughtful observation can round out our initial impressions, expand our view of a situation, and press the pause button to prevent a potentially harmful reflexive response.

In Clara's case, taking a moment to *watch* won't be easy. She has a long history of fraught interactions with her sister, and her first reaction is to feel insulted. Frances's comment hurts, because Clara feels some shame about her inability to reach Angela, her inability to connect. Her knee-jerk response might be to snap and sarcastically reply with something like, "Thanks for the awesome advice, now how about you mind your own business!" From there, an argument might ensue. Another response might be to say nothing, keep her feelings inside, run over the comment again and again in her mind, and harbor her resentment and shame until she's furious by the time of the next family get-together.

Watch refers to the entire situation: the environment, the person you're interacting with, and you. Is the situation unusual or common? What typically happens next? What have I not considered that might be an important part of what is unfolding?

For Clara, this might mean thinking about how her sister experiences these family functions. Maybe Frances is not comfortable around Clara because Clara has always been "the cool aunt." Or there could be some stress in Frances's life, such as concern about their mother's health, that has nothing to do with what's happening in the moment. This *watch* phase might take some time and even extend over the next hour or so. Clara might let Frances's comment go in the moment and then ask her mother what she thought was going on there. If she did this, she might learn that Frances has been having fights with her husband, or that she's feeling pressured at work. This kind of consideration is not meant to excuse behavior, but simply to flesh out the context of what's happening. Context is incredibly valuable. It never hurts to take in as much information as possible, beyond what you notice right away.

The curiosity that we muster during the *watch* phase also includes curiosity about your own emerging reactions—how you're feeling, and why. You might notice what's happening in your body, that your heart is beating faster, that you're pursing your lips or gritting your teeth (signs of anger). You might notice an impulse to lash out or to hide yourself because you feel ashamed. Becoming more conscious of how you react and what you might be about to do can help you ride that wave of emotion rather than having it crash over you.

This leads us to the second stage, which is a critical turning point in response to stress: *interpreting* what the situation means for you.

Stage Two: Interpret (Naming the Stakes)

It is in this stage where things often go wrong.

Interpreting is something we are all doing, all the time, whether we know it or not; we look around at the world, at what is happening to us, and we assess *why* those things are happening, and what it *means* for us. Of course, we build this assessment on reality, but reality is not always so clear-cut. Each of us perceives and interprets a situation in our own way, so what we see as "reality" may not be what other people see. One of the major pitfalls is thinking that a situation is all about us; it rarely is.

If you want to understand a situation as clearly as possible, you first need to make sense of what's at stake for you. Emotion is usually a sign that there is something important going on for you; if there wasn't, you wouldn't be feeling anything. An emotion could be related to an important goal in your life, a particular insecurity, or a relationship you cherish. Asking the question, *Why am I getting emotional?* is a good way to figure out what's at stake for you. If you see the stakes clearly, you may be able to interpret the situation more skillfully.

Bob refers to this stage as "filling in the blank." Because our observation of a situation is rarely complete, we often jump to conclusions about what we don't know. Many situations are ambiguous and unclear, and it is on this canvas of ambiguity that we can project all sorts of ideas. If we've only done a quick-and-dirty job of observing in the *watch* stage, we probably don't have all the information we could have about what's really going on, which leads to hasty conclusions.

In Clara's case, she might think, *Why did that comment make me so mad? Is this about my sister, or about my difficulties with Angela, or just about Angela? My feelings are incredibly strong—why is this so important to me?*

Considering her sister, she might think, *Is Frances doing this on purpose to hurt me or is she doing this because she really thinks she's going to help Angela? Is it because she resents that I don't encourage her to be more involved in Angela's life? Is it possible that she doesn't feel valued in the family as the elder sister who has useful advice?*

When we fill in the blanks, we sometimes make mountains out of molehills. It often happens that we snag on negative aspects of a stressor and turn something small and manageable into something enormous and overwhelming.

Just asking the question—*What is it I'm assuming here?*—can bring what looks like a mountain closer into line with its molehill reality. Assumptions are the source of an incredible amount of misunderstanding. As the old saying goes, *Never assume, because when you assume, you make an ass of u and me.*

But it's also possible to err in the opposite direction and make true mountains into molehills, as in the example of Abigail, who found a lump in her breast and told no one. If we're trying to minimize or avoid thinking about a big problem, we might ignore it entirely.

The important thing in the *interpret* stage is to expand our understanding beyond our initial automatic perception. To consider more perspectives, even if those perspectives are uncomfortable. To ask, *What might I be overlooking here?*

Again, this is a place where some attention to our own emotions can be helpful. When you feel a pulse of fear, a pulse of anger, or a sinking feeling in your stomach, think of it as a signal to inject some healthy curiosity into the situation, to ponder not only the stressor itself, but also your own emotional reality: *Why am I feeling this way? Where are these emotions coming from? What is really at stake? What is so challenging for me about this situation?*

Stage Three: Select (Choosing from the Options)

You've made a point to *watch*, you've *interpreted* (and then reinterpreted) the situation and expanded your view; now the question becomes, *What should I do?*

When we are under stress, we sometimes find ourselves reacting before we have considered our options, or even considered that we might *have* any options. Slowing down can allow us to consider possibilities and think about the likelihood of success for those possibilities: *Given what's at stake and the resources at my disposal, what can I do in this situation? What would be a good outcome here? And what is the likelihood that things will go well if I respond this way instead of that way?*

It's in the *select* stage that we clarify what our goals are and what resources we have at our disposal. *What do I want to accomplish? How best can I accomplish that goal? Do I have strengths that can help me (e.g., humor and an ability to take the edge off heated conversations), or weaknesses that could hurt me (e.g., a tendency to snap when criticized)?*

Let's say that Clara has talked to her mother and gotten some perspective. She realizes that Frances really is worried about Angela, but Frances doesn't understand that the situation is different than with Frances's own kids. Clara realizes she has more than one goal here: she wants to maintain a positive relationship with her sister, protect her daughter from criticism, and also feel good about her ability as a mother.

So now Clara thinks about what she should do; the options, and the likelihood that each option will lead to a positive outcome. She worries that if she does nothing, Frances will continue criticizing her child and blaming Clara for not being a good enough parent. So she decides to say something. But how? And when? They often rib each other, but Clara doesn't feel like joking when her feelings are hurt, and she knows any joke will sound passive-aggressive and make things worse. So she decides to wait until she and Frances are alone, and talk to her then. In thinking about this talk, she realizes that Frances might actually be a helpful sounding board for some of her struggles with Angela, but she definitely does not want Frances to give advice.

Clara has to choose among options at this stage. One response may not (and probably will not) be the end of it. No one approach by itself is likely to be effective in addressing all the challenges in a complicated situation or in a relationship across time. Clara may try multiple strategies with her sister in the coming months. And, of course, circumstances change; her sister may have some highly visible and difficult parenting challenges of her own, and this might change how Clara responds to her sister.

Selecting a strategy is highly personal. Cultural norms and our individual values play important roles here. Confronting someone directly is considered bad manners in some cultures, while in others it is considered mature and authentic. Often, it comes down to intuition honed by experience—what feels like the best way to respond to this situation, in this moment.

Using the W.I.S.E.R. model as a guide for responding to a stressor may at times be difficult. The stressor may happen fast and there may not be time to slow down your response. Or the source of stress may recur and evolve over time, so you may need to revisit these stages as the situation changes. The key is to try to slow things down where you can, zoom in, and move from a fully automatic response to a more considered and purposeful response that aligns with who you are and what you are seeking to accomplish.

Stage Four: Engage (Implementing With Care)

Now it's time to respond as skillfully as possible, to *engage* the strategy you've selected. If you've taken some time to observe and interpret the situation, and if you've made some effort to consider the possibilities and their likelihood of success, your response is more likely to succeed. But the proof of the pudding is in the eating. Even the most logical response can fail if we do a poor job implementing that strategy. Practice—either in our minds or running it by a trusted confidant—can help. Chances of success also increase if we first reflect on what we do well and what we don't do so well. Some of us are funny, and we know that people respond well to our sense of humor. Some of us are more soft-spoken, and we know that quiet discussion in private settings is more comfortable for us.

Clara gets up the nerve to say something when she and Frances have cleared the dishes together and they are alone in the kitchen. She's direct, and calm; her emotions are still there but they are more in the background. At first it goes well; Frances is apologetic for offering unsolicited advice (she's been thinking about her comment, too, and felt bad for how it came out). The two of them agree that they both want what's best for Angela, and Clara shares some recent problems, which Frances understands. Then Clara says something about Angela being her own person and not being like Frances's kids (it sounded so good in her head!) and the situation turns quickly. Frances really has been under a lot of stress at work and arguing more than usual with her husband, so Clara's comment hits a raw nerve. They start to argue again, and then are interrupted by their mother.

"I kind of like it when you fight," their mother says.

"Like it? Why?"

"Because it reminds me of what you were like when you were younger, and I feel like I'm 35 again."

They laugh. But soon that feeling wears off, and the two sisters leave the barbecue with strong emotions and things still not fully resolved.

Stage Five: Reflect (Monday Morning Quarterbacking)

How did that work out? Did I make things better or worse? Have I learned something new about the challenge I'm facing and about the best response?

Reflecting on our response to a challenge can yield dividends for the future. It's in learning from experience that we truly grow wiser. We can do this not only for something that just happened, but for events both big and small that have happened in the past and linger in our memories. Take a look at the worksheet below and consider using it to *reflect* on an incident or situation that's troubling you.

WATCH
Did I face the problem directly or try to avoid it?
Did I take time to get an accurate assessment of the situation?
Did I talk with the people involved?
Did I consult with others to get their understanding of what happened?

INTERPRET
Did I recognize how I felt and what was at stake for me in this situation?
Was I willing to acknowledge my role in the situation?
Have I focused too much on what is going on in my own head and not enough on what is going on around me?
Are there alternative ways of understanding what is going on in this situation?

SELECT
Was I clear about the outcome I wanted?
Did I consider all the available options for responding?
Did I do a good job identifying resources available to help me?
Did I weigh the pros and cons of different strategies to achieve my goals?
Did I choose the tools that would work best in meeting the current challenge?
Did I reflect on IF or WHEN I should do something about the situation?
Did I consider who else could be involved in solving the problem or meeting the challenge?

ENGAGE
Did I practice my response or run it by a trusted confidant to increase the likelihood that it would succeed?
Did I take steps that are realistic for me?
Did I evaluate progress and was I willing to adjust as needed?
What steps did I rush through or mess up or skip over? What did I do well?

In light of all I've just reflected on, how would I do things differently next time? What have I learned?

Don't worry if this list of questions, or even the W.I.S.E.R. model in general, seems like too much to think about at once. Many of the steps in the W.I.S.E.R. model may be things you already do instinctively, and 90 percent of everyday life doesn't require this kind of reflection. Think of the model and this list of questions as a kind of coaching tool for that final 10 percent of life when you feel stuck, or you notice yourself behaving in ways that don't serve you well.

When it's all over, the consideration of what happened, and why, helps us to see things we may have missed, and helps us understand the causes and effects of these emotional cascades that may have escaped our notice. If we're going to learn from our experience and do better next time, we have to do more than just live through it. We have to reflect. In doing so, when we find ourselves in the heat of a similar moment next time, we may be able to take that extra split second to consider the situation, clarify our goals, consider options for responding to it, and move the needle of our lives in the right direction.

GETTING UNSTUCK

The W.I.S.E.R. model is most straightforward when it is applied to discrete relationship challenges. But stress comes in all varieties, and many involve more chronic patterns in our relationships. Sometimes we encounter similar things over and over in a relationship, the same arguments, the same annoyances, the same sequence of unhelpful responses. We end up feeling that we are not moving forward, and we can't imagine getting out of our current rut. The two of us, Bob and Marc, refer to this feeling with the highly scientific name of *stuckness*.

We see this both in our Harvard Study participants and among people who come to us seeking psychotherapy. People often feel stuck in their lives and may not be able to articulate fully why they feel that way. They may find themselves having the same disagreements with a partner over and over, no longer able to have even a simple conversation that does not get heated. At work, it might feel like a boss is frequently micromanaging and finding fault, leading to a sense of worthlessness that can be difficult to overcome. (In fact, work relationships that fall into a rut are some of the most vexing. More on that in Chapter Nine.)

For example, John Marsden from Chapter Two found himself deeply lonely in his early 80s, in part because he and his wife were locked in a repetitive cycle of not giving each other what they most needed—affection and support.

> Q: Do you ever go to your wife when you're upset?
>
> A: No. Definitely not. I would get no sympathy. I would be told that it's a sign of weakness. I mean I can't tell you the negative signals I get all day it's just . . . it's so destructive.

John was thinking about the reality of his life—about real conversations with his partner. But without realizing it, he was also constructing that reality. His isolation from his wife became a self-fulfilling prophecy. He saw every new encounter with her as proof of his theory: *She doesn't want to be close to me, I can't trust her with my feelings.*

As the modern Buddhist teacher Shohaku Okumura writes, "The world we live in is the world we create."

As in many Buddhist teachings, there is a double meaning there. Humans physically create the world we live in, but at every moment we are also creating a picture of the world in our minds by telling stories to ourselves—individually and collectively—that may or may not be true.

No two relationships are the same, but one person will often get stuck in similar places in different relationships. The old saying, "We're always fighting the last battle," is very true. We tend to think that the thing that happened to us before is about to happen again, whether that is the case or not.

At their core, feelings of stuckness come from patterns in our lives. Some patterns help us navigate life efficiently and quickly, but others may lead us to respond in ways that don't serve us well. These patterns may include spending time with the wrong people—the wrong friends, and even the wrong partners. Far from being random, these patterns often reflect areas of preoccupation and struggles from our past, which in a way feel like home. They are like a set of familiar dance steps that we fall into. A familiar sensation, even if it's negative, is activated in a conversation with someone, and there is a kind of comfort in that familiarity. *Oh here it is again, I know this dance.*

Most of us feel a certain amount of stuckness to some degree, so the question is really about the strength of that feeling. Is it consistently diminishing your quality of life? Is it pervasive, shaping many or most areas of your daily experience?

Bob was stuck in a pattern himself earlier in his life. He dated a series of women, and his friends were consistently surprised at the partners he was choosing. The relationships kept souring. Feeling stuck, he went into psychotherapy, and in describing each of these failed relationships to his therapist, he saw that these failures weren't coincidences or a string of bad luck. His therapist helped him realize that he'd been choosing the same type of person over and over again—a type of person with whom he was not compatible. Getting honest perspectives on your life from people you trust can be very illuminating in your effort to become unstuck. Such trusted observers will almost certainly see things that you can't.

You may also be able to do something like this yourself by asking, *If someone else was telling me this story, what would I think? What would I tell them?* This kind of self-distanced reflection can shed new light on old stories.

Realizing that you may not be seeing the whole picture is a big first step in breaking free of mental patterns that lock us in. The Zen master Shunryu Suzuki taught that it is a positive thing to approach some situations in life as if you've never lived them before. "In the beginner's mind there are many possibilities," he wrote, "but in the expert's mind there are few." We all feel like experts when it comes to our own lives, and the challenge is to stay open to the possibility that there is more we can learn about ourselves—to allow ourselves to be beginners.

RELATIONSHIPS, ADAPTATION, AND THE END OF THE WORLD

When the Covid-19 pandemic struck the world in 2020, the social isolation, financial strain, and constant worry was an enormous shock to societies all over the globe. As the pandemic and lockdowns continued, isolation and anxiety around the world surged. Stress levels went through the roof. It was, by many measures, a challenge on a scale that the world had not experienced since World War II.

When the pandemic began, we went back to our Study records to read once more what our original Study members told us about how they got through big life crises. They had grown up in the Great Depression, and most of the college men had served in World War II. What most of them recalled was that in order to survive these great crises, they leaned on their most important relationships. The men who fought in the war talked about the bonds they formed with their fellow soldiers and how important those bonds were, not just for their safety but also for their sanity. After the war, many talked about how important it was to be able to share at least part of their experiences with their wives. In fact, those who did so were more likely to stay married. The support they got from others during those hard times, and later in processing them, was crucial. And we find that today.

The pandemic froze our lives, locked us in with those we live with, kept us apart from the friends and coworkers we were accustomed to seeing every day. We never signed up to be with our spouses and children 24/7, but we had to make do. Many older adults never dreamed that they'd be separated from their precious grandchildren for more than an entire year.

Flexibility became more important than ever. To survive we had to give each other space, cut each other slack. If we needed distance from a spouse, it may not have been because there was something wrong with the relationship but because these were abnormal times.

Sadly, Covid-19 won't be the last global catastrophe, or the last pandemic. These things will continue to come . . . and go. That's the nature of life.

The Harvard Study teaches us that it's crucial to lean on those relationships that can hold us up when things go sideways, just as the Study families did during the Great Depression, World War II, and the Great Recession in 2008. Through the Covid-19 pandemic, that meant staying in touch, in a purposeful way, with people who were now suddenly distant from us. Sending that text, setting up a video chat, making a phone call. Not just thinking of a distant friend but reaching out. It meant being patient with the people we love and asking for help when we needed it. The same will be true for the next crisis, and the next.

For Marc, the idea that relationships help us navigate major challenges is quite personal.

In December of 1939, at the same time that Arlie Bock was interviewing Harvard College sophomores in his mission to figure out what makes people healthy, Marc's father, Robert Schulz, then 10 years old, was on a passenger ship with his older sister, crossing the Atlantic Ocean. Born to a Jewish family in Hamburg, they'd fled Nazi Germany, and arrived in the United States with only the clothes on their backs, two small suitcases, and no clear plan.

But they were alive. And for one major reason: Marc's grandmother's natural habit of forming deep connections with people.

Marc's father remembers an idyllic early life as a child in Hamburg. Even as his family navigated his father's death at a young age, he was surrounded by family and friends. Life was good. His family's textile business was thriving, and he was into gymnastics and playing the piano. Marc heard him talk often about the beauty of Hamburg, the lake at the center of the city, and especially marzipan, a sweet, almond-flavored German treat, a staple of his early childhood.

He had a charmed life back then, he always said.

But things began to change as the Nazis consolidated power and began their campaigns against Jews. Etched in his memory was a particularly scary day and night in November of 1938 when he was nine years old. During the evening of terror that would come to be known as *Kristallnacht*, or "Crystal Night," many Jewish homes, businesses, and synagogues in his neighborhood were destroyed or burned to the ground. The next day, the Gestapo came to his school and rounded up many of the Jewish teachers and students.

As deportations and detentions of Jews were being conducted all over the city, Marc's grandmother reached out to close friends of hers, a German family that ran a dairy down the street. They agreed to hide Marc's father and his family in the basement of the dairy. Without the combination of this kindness and a great deal of luck, they would not have survived.

Even to this day, Marc stays in touch with the descendants of that family in Germany, who tell the same story but from the perspective of their parents and grandparents, who'd made a decision in the moment to protect their friends at grave risk to themselves. It was an act of kindness that could have cost them their lives. Without them, Marc would not exist.

ACCEPTING THE BIG RISK

The question for us in our daily lives is: When we confront personal or global challenges, when people hurt us, or when we find that we have hurt others . . . what do we *do*?

Human beings are mysterious, wonderful, dangerous creatures. We are at once vulnerable and incredibly resilient. We have the capacity for creating both magnificent beauty and vast destruction.

That's the big picture. But if we zoom in a little bit and focus on the life of a single person . . . your life, let's say . . . and even the small events and stresses in your life, the complexity of who we are remains.

If you're like most people, you struggle, at least sometimes, to understand the people in your life—from those you love most to those you barely know. It's difficult to really connect with other people and know them. It's difficult to love and to be loved. It's difficult to keep from pushing love away.

But making the effort can bring joy, novelty, safety—and sometimes it can even be lifesaving. Slowing down, attempting to see difficult situations clearly, and cultivating positive relationships can help us manage the waves, whether they come from a political crisis, a strange virus that travels around the globe, a moment of reckoning about who we really are, or a rush of anger at a family barbecue. Our initial, automatic responses are not the only ways we can respond. Recognizing this can allow us to pause in the midst of challenge, in the midst of our own bad luck, our own repeating problems, even our own mistakes, and chart a path forward.

In the coming chapters, we will talk about applying the ideas we've discussed so far to particular kinds of relationships. Every type of relationship is a little bit different; family relationships are different from work relationships, which are different from marriages, which are different from friendships. Of course, sometimes these categories overlap. Our family members might also be our coworkers, and our siblings might also be our best friends. Still, broad categories can be helpful to consider, while still remembering that each relationship is unique and requires its own kind of attention and adaptation. In the next chapter, we'll start close to the heart, with the person beside you.

THE PERSON BESIDE YOU

How Intimate Relationships Shape Our Lives

When we were children, we used to think that when we were grown-up we would no longer be vulnerable. But to grow up is to accept vulnerability. . . . To be alive is to be vulnerable.

Madeleine L'Engle

Harvard Study Questionnaire, 1979

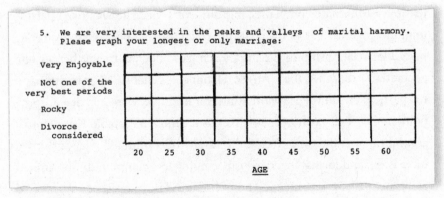

5. We are very interested in the peaks and valleys of marital harmony. Please graph your longest or only marriage:

Very Enjoyable								
Not one of the very best periods								
Rocky								
Divorce considered								

AGE: 20 25 30 35 40 45 50 55 60

In Plato's *Symposium*, Aristophanes gives a speech about the origin of human beings. In the beginning, he says, every human had four legs, four arms, and two heads. They were strong and ambitious creatures. Zeus, in order to diminish their fearsome powers, split them all down the middle. Now, walking on only two legs, every human is in search of their other half. " 'Love,' " Plato says, "is the name for our pursuit of wholeness, for our desire to be complete."

After thousands of years, this idea still resonates.

"Jean is my better half," Dill Carson, one of the inner-city Boston participants, told the Harvard Study when asked about his wife. "Every evening we sit down and have a glass of wine. It's a kind of ritual, I don't feel the day is complete without it. We talk about the things we're feeling and what's going on. If we had an argument, we'll talk about that. We talk about plans, about the kids. It kind of rounds out the day, smooths over the rough edges. If I had to do it all over again, I'd marry the same woman, without a doubt."

My better half . . . It's a sentiment that a number of Harvard Study participants expressed when asked about their partners. The deepest and most positive intimate connections often gave participants a feeling, as Plato was suggesting, of balance and unity.

Unfortunately, there is no universal formula for happy partnerships, happy romances, happy marriages, no single magical key that can unlock the joys of intimate companionship for everyone. The way two "halves" might fit together varies from culture to culture, and of course from one particular relationship to the next. Even from one era to another, or one generation to another, the forms of relationships change. Most of the original participants in the Harvard Study, for example, were married at some point in their life, partly because this was the most acceptable expression of commitment at the time. Today, the variety of committed relationships is increasing, and formal marriage is becoming less common. In the United States in 2020, 51 percent of all households did not consist of any married couples. In 1950, the number was closer to 20 percent. But a change in form doesn't necessarily mean a change in feeling; human beings remain much the same. Even within the range of seemingly "traditional" marriages there can be a lot of variation. Love comes in all shapes and sizes.

Take James Brewer, one of the Study's college participants. He came from a small town in Indiana, and when he first arrived at Harvard he was an intelligent but still naive young man with little life experience. He told the Study he could not understand the idea of "heterosexuality." To him it made no sense that anyone should be restricted to having sex with only one gender—as far as he was concerned, beauty was beauty, and love was love. He was attracted to both men and women; shouldn't everybody feel that way? He was open about this idea with his friends and fellow students until he began to encounter resistance, and then significant prejudice, at which point he began to hide his sexuality. Soon after college, he married Maryanne, whom he deeply loved and who loved him, and they had kids and lived a full life together. But in 1978, after thirty-one years of marriage, Maryanne died of breast cancer, at the age of 57.

When the Study asked James why he thought their marriage had lasted so long, he wrote,

> We survived because we shared so very much. She read important parts of good books to me. We talked of castles and kings, of cabbages, and many other things. We looked and compared notes on what we saw. . . . We enjoyed eating together, seeing places together, sleeping together. . . . Our parties, our best parties, were spontaneous ones that we created for just the two of us, often as surprises for each other.

Three years after Maryanne's death, a Harvard Study interviewer visited James in his home. During the visit James asked the interviewer to follow him as he went into a brightly lit room chattering with birds. Beside the windows were a few cages, and in the middle of the room, several rope lattices and artificial trees. The birds alighted on him as he opened their cages and fed them. They were his wife's birds, he told the interviewer, still so grief-stricken that he couldn't manage to say her name. Asked about his current love life, he said that he'd had some short-lived relationships, that many people thought of him as gay, and while he wasn't currently in a relationship, he hadn't given up on the possibility. "I suppose eventually someone will come along and touch my heart," he said.

As anyone who has loved another person knows, the pursuit of intimate connection is not without hazards: by opening ourselves to the joy of loving and being loved, we risk being hurt. The closer we feel to another person, the more vulnerable we become. Yet we continue to take that risk.

This chapter wades into the deep end of intimacy and the effect intimate connection has on well-being. We encourage you to see everything we offer in the coming pages through the lens of your own personal experiences, and to try to uncover some of the reasons behind both the successes and the challenges you've had in intimate relationships. As the lives of our Harvard Study participants show, recognizing and understanding your emotions, and how those emotions affect your intimate partner—the person beside you—can have both subtle and sweeping impacts on your life.

INTIMACY, AND ALLOWING OURSELVES TO BE KNOWN

We asked Study participants and their partners a set of questions about intimacy again and again over many decades. This allowed us to see each unique trajectory of feeling—affection, tension, and love—from a relationship's beginnings to its very end. These relationships ran the gamut from brief and fiery to long and sleepy, and everything in between. Let's look at one of those that's in between:

Joseph Cichy and his wife, Olivia, married in 1948 and remained married until Olivia passed away in 2007 just after their fifty-ninth wedding anniversary. Their marriage is representative of a strong partnership, and the ways that two people can support each other over the duration of a life. But their partnership is representative for another reason, too: it was far from perfect.

Over the years, whenever the Study checked in with Joseph, he reported that he felt good about his life. He had a career he liked, three wonderful kids, and a "peaceful" relationship with his wife. In 2008, we asked their daughter, Lily, to reflect on her childhood and she told the Study that her parents were about as calm as a married couple could be. She couldn't remember them having a single argument.

Joseph had given a similar account to the Study across many years. "I am as easy to get along with as anyone who ever lived," he triumphantly told the Study in 1967 when he was 46 years old. He loved his wife, Olivia, just as she was, he said; there was nothing he would change about her. He gave his children the same respect he would give to anyone, offering guidance when they asked for it, but not trying to control them. In his work as a businessman, he did his best to listen to the perspectives of others before offering his own view of a situation. "The only form of persuasion that works is to empathize," he said.

It was a philosophy that served Joseph well his entire life. He enjoyed listening to people and learning about their experiences. We've been making the case that understanding how others feel and think is beneficial to us in our relationships, and Joseph is a great example of this. But for everyone who was close to Joseph, this interest in people and ability to listen coexisted with a problem: he was afraid of opening *himself* to others, even the people he loved.

And this included his wife, Olivia.

"The greatest stress in our marriage isn't conflict," Joseph told the Study. "It's Olivia's frustration about my unwillingness to let her get inside me. She feels shut out." She was honest with him about how much this concerned her, and Joseph was well aware of her concern, telling the Study on several occasions that Olivia often told him how difficult he was to truly know. "I'm self-sufficient," he said. "My biggest weakness is not leaning on anybody. I'm just made that way."

Joseph was tuned in enough to other people that he could see and articulate their difficulty with him, but he could never get past a core, deeply rooted fear that is not uncommon: he didn't want to be a burden, or to feel anything but fully independent. Though he attended Harvard, Joseph came from humble beginnings, and told the Study that he learned the value of self-sufficiency as a child on his family farm, where he spent days on end operating a horse-drawn plow alone. His mother and father were busy with their own work on the farm, and Joseph was expected to take care of himself. As an adult he believed he should handle any problems he encountered—emotional or otherwise—on his own. He didn't see anything wrong with that.

In 2008, his daughter Lily, who was in her 50s, told a Study interviewer that she still lamented this philosophy. Her father was always there for practical support when she needed him, and she felt she could count on him at any time of the day or night (and in fact, she did count on him; he helped her through a difficult marriage and some of the most trying times of her life). But she never felt that she fully knew him.

At the age of 72, when asked about his relationship to his wife, Joseph told the Study that the marriage was stable, but that there was also a sense of disconnection between them. "There's nothing pulling us apart," he said, "but we're not bound together."

Joseph had decided as a young man that in his relationships, two things were more important than anything else: keeping the peace, and being self-sufficient. It was important to him that his life and his family's life be stable above all else. This wasn't necessarily wrong; his life, by most measures, was a good one. He loved his family, and they were all very loyal to each other. Joseph was conducting his life in the way that felt safe, and to the extent his approach prevented strife, it worked for him. It's not bad to have a marriage where there's little disagreement. But are there costs to *always* keeping the peace? By being so protective of his inner experience, and so selective about what he shared—by not being daring enough to open himself up—was Joseph denying both himself and Olivia the full benefits of an intimate connection?

Many of us have someone like this in our lives; we should remember it's not necessarily a sign that they don't care. But Olivia, at least, felt a sense of incompleteness, because the keystone of intimacy is the feeling of knowing someone and of *being* known. In fact, the word *intimacy* comes from the Latin *intimare*: to make known. Intimate knowledge of another person is a feature of romantic love, but it's also more than that. It's a quintessential piece of the human experience, and it begins long before our first kiss, long before we consider marriage, in the very earliest days of life.

INTIMATE ATTACHMENT: THE STRANGE SITUATION

From the moment we are born we begin seeking close connections, both physical and emotional, to other people. We begin life as helpless creatures, dependent on others for our very survival. Almost everything we encounter as infants is intensely novel and potentially threatening, so it's essential that we establish a strong connection to at least one other person from the very first days of life. Being close to our mothers or fathers or grandparents or aunties is comforting and provides a refuge from danger. As we grow, we can explore the world beyond our comfort zone knowing that we have a safe place to go if things get scary. The simplicity and clarity of the young child's situation provides a great opportunity to observe the fundamentals of human emotional connection. This period of life vividly displays some core truths about close emotional bonds that are relevant for adults as well as children.

In the 1970s, Mary Ainsworth, a psychologist, designed a laboratory procedure to help reveal how babies respond to the world around them and the people on whom they are most dependent. It's known as the "Strange Situation," and it has proved so useful over the decades that it's still employed in research today, more than fifty years later. The key elements of it work like this:

A baby, usually between 9 and 18 months old, accompanied by her primary caregiver, is introduced to a room with some toys in it. After spending a short time in the room interacting with the caregiver and playing with the toys, a stranger enters. At first the stranger minds her own business, lets the child get used to her presence, and then tries to connect with the baby. A short time later, the caregiver leaves the room.

Now the baby finds herself in a strange place, with a strange person, and no one with whom she feels close. Often the baby will immediately show signs of discomfort and begin to cry.

A short time later, the caregiver returns.

What happens next is a key reason for the experiment. The child has encountered a strange situation, experienced some stress, and now her caregiver has returned. The researchers have deliberately disrupted the infant's sense of safety and connection—albeit briefly—and the child needs to reestablish these. How will she respond? The way the infant attempts to stay connected to the person on whom she depends for survival—her *attachment style*—is believed to reveal how the child views her caregiver and also herself.

A SECURE BASE

Each of us has a particular way of staying connected to a person we need. Attachment styles are relevant not just to understanding early childhood, but also to understanding how we manage relationships throughout our lives.

It is normal for children to get upset when a caregiver leaves, and in fact this is what the healthy, well-adjusted child does. When the caregiver returns, the child will immediately seek contact, and upon receiving it, calm down and return to a state of equilibrium. The child seeks contact during this "reunion" because she views her caregiver as a source of love and safety and also feels *deserving* of that love. A child who displays this sort of attachment behavior is considered *securely attached*.

But infants who feel less securely attached cope with that insecurity in two different ways: by expressing anxiety or avoidance. More anxious infants will seek immediate contact when the caregiver returns to them, but have trouble being soothed. Avoidant children, on the other hand, may appear on the surface to be unconcerned about the caregiver's presence. They may show little outward distress when the caregiver leaves the room, and may not seek comfort when the caregiver returns. They sometimes even turn away from the caregiver during the reunion. Parents may take this to mean that the child doesn't care. But appearances in such cases can be deceiving. Attachment researchers theorize that these avoidant children *do* care when the caregiver leaves, but they have learned not to make too many demands on their caregiver. They do this, according to the theory, because they've sensed that expressing their needs may not result in receiving love, and may also drive the caregiver away.

In real life, children encounter variations on the Strange Situation repeatedly—when they're dropped off at daycare and then picked up at the end of the day, for example—and each of these encounters shapes their expectations about future relationships. They develop a sense of how likely it is that others will be helpful, and also a judgment about how deserving they are of support.

Adult life is, in some fundamental ways, a real-world, highly complex version of the Strange Situation. Like every child who has been separated from their parent, each of us longs for a sense of security, or what psychologists call a *secure base of attachment*. A child may feel threatened because her mother is not in the room, and an adult may feel threatened by a frightening health diagnosis; both benefit from a sense that someone is there for them.

But attachment security exists on a spectrum for adults as well, and many of us are not fully secure in our attachments. Some of us may cling to others during times of stress yet have difficulty finding the comfort we seek, while others, like Joseph Cichy, may avoid closeness because we fear, deep down, that if we become a burden to others, we will drive them away. Or we may not be convinced that we are fully lovable. And yet we still need connection. Life becomes more complex as we age, *but the benefits that come from having secure connections continue through every phase of life.*

Henry and Rosa Keane, from Chapter One, are a shining example of two people with secure connections. Every time they faced a difficulty together—from one of their children contracting polio, to Henry being laid off, to the task of facing their own mortality—they were able to turn to each other for support, comfort, and courage.

The sequence for both babies and adults is often similar: a stress or difficulty disturbs our sense of security, and we seek to restore that sense. If we're lucky we are able to do this by gaining comfort from those who are close to us, and we return to equilibrium.

In our last interview with them, sitting at their kitchen table, Henry and Rosa kept physically reaching out for each other, especially when answering difficult questions about future health challenges and their own mortality. Through most of the interview, they were holding hands.

That simplest of gestures—holding a partner's hand—is a helpful portal into the world of adult intimate attachment. In the Strange Situation, when a securely attached child seeks her caregiver and is comforted by a hug, there are physiological and psychological benefits. Her body and her emotions are calmed. Is the same true for adults? What's happening exactly when someone holds our hand?

LOVING CONTACT: THE EQUIVALENT OF A DRUG

James Coan ventured into the world of attachment research by accident. He had wanted to know what was happening in the brains of people suffering from post-traumatic stress disorder (a mental health condition characterized by flashbacks, nightmares, and worries about a traumatic event), and he was scanning their brains for clues. With a better understanding of their brain activity, he hoped, new treatments could be devised and their suffering could be eased. One of his study participants happened to be a Vietnam War veteran with intense combat experience who refused to participate in the research without his wife in the room. Coan was eager for his participation and was happy to make accommodations that allowed the study to continue, so the man's wife sat beside him while he lay in the fMRI (brain scanning) machine.

MRI machines can be loud, and when the test began the man became agitated and didn't want to continue. His wife, sitting beside him, sensed his agitation and instinctively took his hand in hers. This had a calming effect on him, and he was able to go on.

Coan was intrigued by this effect, and when the study was over, he developed a new brain imaging study to see if he could find some neural evidence for what had happened.

Participants in the new experiment were put into the fMRI machine and shown one of two slides. A red slide meant there was a 20 percent chance they would receive a small electrical shock. A blue slide meant they would not receive a shock.

The participants were divided into three groups: the first group had no one in the room with them during the experiment. The second group held the hand of a complete stranger. The third group held the hand of a spouse.

The results were crystal-clear: holding hands with someone they felt close to calmed the activity in the fear centers of participants' brains, and diminished their anxiety. But perhaps most remarkable, holding hands with someone they felt close to actually diminished the *amount of pain* participants said they felt when they received a shock. There was also a benefit to holding the hand of a stranger, but the effect was so pronounced for intimate partners (particularly those in more satisfied relationships) that it led Coan to conclude that holding a loved one's hand during a medical procedure had the same effect as a mild anesthetic. Study participants' relationships were affecting their bodies in real time.

MORE THAN A FEELING

Relationships live inside of us. The mere thought of a person who is important to us can generate hormones and other chemicals that travel through our blood and affect our hearts, our brains, and numerous other body systems. These effects can span a lifetime. As we noted in Chapter One, using data from the Harvard Study, George Vaillant found that marital happiness at age 50 was a better predictor of good physical health in late life than age 50 cholesterol level.

Coan was able to analyze the effect of intimate connection on a person's brain in the lab, but we obviously can't (yet) put ourselves into an fMRI machine while we're on a first date, or when we're having an argument with a partner in a parking lot. Luckily, at the very root of all intimate attachment, regardless of our age, there is a different kind of diagnostic tool that each of us can access just by paying attention:

Emotion.

In any situation in life, emotions are a signal that there are matters of significance to us at play, and they are especially revealing when it comes to intimate relationships. If we take some time to pause and examine that seemingly simple thing, *how we feel*, we can develop an invaluable life tool: the ability to look beneath the surface of our relationships. Our emotions can point us to hidden truths about our wishes and fears, our expectations about how others should behave, and the reasons we view our partners the way we do.

Imagine it this way: when scuba divers descend into a body of water, they have depth indicators on their wrists. But they can also feel the depth in their bodies. The deeper they go, the more pressure they feel.

Emotions are a kind of depth indicator for a relationship. Most of the time we are swimming near the surface of life, interacting with our partners and going about the daily business of living. The underlying emotional currents are buried a bit deeper, in the dark of the water. When we experience a strong emotion, positive or negative—a sudden welling-up of gratitude, or a surge of anger at being misunderstood—it's an indication of something deeper. If we make an effort to pause in these moments, to *watch* and *interpret*, as we've suggested in our W.I.S.E.R. model of interaction (Chapter Six), we can begin to see more clearly the things that are important to us, and also what's important to our partners.

NURTURING A BEDROCK OF EMPATHY AND AFFECTION

How important are the emotions that we feel (and express) during interactions with our partners? Can emotions indicate the strength of connection, and the likelihood of a lasting partnership?

We investigated the link between emotion and relationship stability in one of our earliest joint research studies. We brought couples who were married or living together into the lab and videotaped them for eight to ten minutes as they discussed a recent upsetting incident in their relationship. Later the videos were rated for how much each partner expressed specific emotions (for example, affection, anger, humor) and behaviors (for example, "acknowledges partner's perspective").

We specifically asked research assistants who did not have extensive training in psychology to rate the emotions in these videos. Would these untrained observers' natural human ability to recognize how others are feeling be useful in predicting stability in relationships?

Five years later, we checked back with the couples to see how they were doing. Some were still together, some were not. When we set their relationship status beside our research assistants' ratings of emotions in their earlier interactions, we found that the ratings predicted with close to 85 percent accuracy which couples had stayed together. This is consistent with many other studies showing that emotions between partners are a critical indicator of whether intimate relationships thrive or fail. The fact that raters with no special knowledge of psychology could accurately predict relationship strength was significant because it showed that most adults have a facility to accurately read emotions. Most of the raters had not yet experienced deep, longer-term relationships, yet when they looked closely, they could sense important, sometimes subtle emotions and behaviors in the couples. *Emotions drive relationships, and noticing them matters.*

Not every type of emotion is equally predictive of the health of a relationship, however. Some are particularly important, and in our study, two categories of emotion stood out:

Empathy and affection.

The men and women who expressed more affectionate emotions while they were discussing something upsetting with their partner were more likely to be together five years later. Empathic responses from the men were also important. The more that men were tuned in to their partner's feelings, the more they showed interest in understanding their partner, and the more they acknowledged their partner's perspective, the more likely the couple was to stay together. These findings, along with our findings about the importance of empathic effort (discussed in Chapter 5), point to an important idea about intimate relationships: *if a couple can cultivate a bedrock of affection and empathy (meaning curiosity and the willingness to listen), their bond will be more stable and enduring.*

A FEAR OF DIFFERENCES

All kinds of things can cause strong, challenging emotions in intimate relationships. Even positive emotions can be challenging. A great love, because of its importance to us, can become plagued by a great fear of loss.

But one of the most common reasons for strong emotions in a relationship is simple differences between partners. Where there is difference, there may be disagreement, and where there is disagreement there is often emotion.

When differences first arise, they can be alarming. After the initial excitement and euphoria of a new relationship begins to wane, you might start to notice things about your partner that worry you. Sometimes it might be Big-D Differences (like whether or not to have kids) that warrant consideration of whether the relationship is right for both of you. But often it's little-d differences that *seem* big because of the adjustments they require. Maybe one of you likes to joke around in times of stress and the other finds nothing funny about hard times. Or one of you loves to explore new restaurants and the other prefers to cook at home.

When you begin to discover these differences, it's easy to feel threatened. If you're married or living together, you might feel as though the specific life you've always imagined is under threat, but you've come too far to turn back. You might feel trapped, and begin to have thoughts like, *My partner is:*

Selfish

Ignorant

Immoral

Damaged

. . . and the differences can come to look like problems that are hard-wired by background or family. This can seem to be evidence of how in-compatible the two of you are.

Psychologist Dan Wile wrote in his book *After the Honeymoon*:

> After the honeymoon. The very words carry a burden of sadness, as if for a short while we lived in a golden trance of love, and now we've been jolted awake. The fog of early infatuation has lifted and we see our partners for who they are. . . . Immediately comes the thought, "Oh no! Is this the person I'm supposed to spend the rest of my life with?"

Confronted with these emotions, we often (and understandably) think the goal should be to avoid or reduce differences. Joseph Cichy was a master at minimizing difficulties. He lived his entire life doing his best to avoid conflict and smooth over any cracks. And in terms of diminish-ing conflict, it worked. But the result was a marriage with less emotional closeness, less intimacy.

So the question becomes, if a smooth relationship with no conflict is not the path to rich and fulfilling intimacy, but conflict often causes stress, what do we do?

THE DANCE

Early in their marriage, Bob and his wife, Jennifer, used their weekly date night to go to a ballroom dancing class. Most of the other couples were engaged and taking the class to help them on their wedding day. During one class Jennifer, who is a psychologist, wondered: Could each couple's way of dancing together be a window into what their relationship was like? As with new challenges in relationships, new dance moves are sometimes awkward at first, and it takes couples time to learn the steps and to adjust to and accommodate each other. One partner is usually a faster "stepper" or more of a natural than the other, but both make mistakes, both are learning. Could their dancing indicate which couples were capable of tolerating and forgiving mistakes? Could their style of resolving problems in the dance predict whether they'd still be together in five years?

Just as with dancing, the old adage that you have to *learn by doing* is especially apt when it comes to relationships. There is give-and-take, flow and counterflow. There are routines, steps, and improvisations. Most importantly, there are mistakes and missteps. No couple is going to be Fred Astaire and Ginger Rogers the first time they take the floor together. (Even Fred and Ginger needed a lot of practice!) Both partners must learn as they go. These missteps are not failures or signs that dancing together is impossible. Instead, they are opportunities to learn; step *here* instead of *there*. My partner wants to go *this way*—I'll go with him. Now I would like to go *that way*—he'll have to learn to come with me. Yes, we notice the mistakes and those moments when we are not in sync. But the important thing is how both dance partners respond.

The same is true in life. *In the end, what matters most are not the challenges we face in relationships, but how we manage them.*

UNDERVALUED OPPORTUNITIES

One thing both of us, Marc and Bob, know from decades of doing couples therapy is that people in intimate relationships often overlook the opportunities presented by disagreements.

It happens all the time: a couple shows up for their first session, and one partner has a very clear idea of why they are there. It often involves pointing a finger at the other person:

> *He has trouble letting things go.*
> *She needs to work on her anger issues.*
> *He doesn't do his share around the house.*

She never wants to go out, but I don't like sitting around.
He's obsessed with sex (or he's not interested in sex).

Whatever the "problem" is, the implication is clear: *my partner needs to be fixed.* But in reality, there's almost always a deeper, more complex tension within the relationship that the couple has not acknowledged. Discovering that tension usually requires both self-reflection and conversation.

In couples therapy, we assume that there will be disagreements and differences, and we encourage couples to recognize and attempt to understand them. *Disagreements, and the emotions that come with them, are opportunities to revitalize a relationship by revealing those important truths hidden below the surface.*

Two lives, in all of their complexity, are bound to include differences that don't quite fit together. Maybe you feel the need to keep things clean and a pile of dirty dishes causes a flash of frustration, or your partner gets angry at you about your attention to your smartphone, or maybe one of you is often running late and that causes arguments.

"You never put the cap back on the toothpaste tube!" one partner might complain, with an emotional weight that doesn't seem to match the circumstances.

The intense feelings that emerge in recurring arguments, however trivial, often come down to one of a few common, but profound concerns. See if any of these ring a bell:

You don't care about me.
I'm working harder at this than you are.
I'm not sure I can trust you.
I'm afraid I'm going to lose you.
You don't think I'm good enough.
You don't accept me for who I am.

Sifting through the emotions of a disagreement to uncover these fears and worries and feelings of vulnerability—both our partner's and our own—isn't always easy. First we have to allow for the possibility that we are missing what's really going on beneath the surface. Because we have an instinct to protect ourselves, we have a tendency to jump to conclusions without realizing that's what we're doing. Just as we flinch or throw up our hands when a physical object is hurled at us, we tend to flinch and pass judgment when a heavy emotion comes our way.

The cap on the toothpaste tube would never bother me—why does it have to bother you? You're too sensitive!

And just like that, rather than investigating the disagreement and the emotions that come with it, we've taken a hard stance, passed judgment, and decided that the problem is our partner's oversensitivity. This kind of judgment happens instantly in all kinds of situations, from "trivial" disagreements to the biggest issues of love and connection.

Joseph Cichy, for example, couldn't see the full extent of his wife's experience because he was too immersed in his own interpretation. He understood that his resistance to being open bothered her, but he'd already decided that his understanding was the right one. In his mind, he was saving her the trouble of hearing about his personal feelings. Sharing his emotions, he thought, would endanger his peaceful relationship with his wife, and he didn't want to lose her. But in an effort to protect against that vulnerability, he was contributing to the vulnerability that his wife felt. After all, the person she was closest to in the world did not seem to need her as much as she needed him.

He never asked the question, *What would it mean for our relationship if I shared more of my feelings?*

We all have our own vulnerabilities, those fears and worries that cause us to react to disagreements by turning away from them to protect ourselves. These emotions are not easy to face, but the disagreements we have with our partners have the potential to reveal them to us.

MUTUAL VULNERABILITY: A SOURCE OF STRENGTH

When our Second Generation participants spoke of the lowest moments in their lives, a large proportion of those moments were related to intimate relationships. Deep, intimate connections are by their nature incredibly vulnerable situations. When two people who are intimate are in harmony, the effect can be exhilarating, but if the relationship falters, the result can cause intense emotional pain, feelings of betrayal, and critical self-examination. As one of our Second Generation participants, Aimee, told the Study:

> My first husband is from Texas and we moved there after meeting in Arizona. We lived in a small town raising our daughters, but my husband worked in Dallas, so he had to spend nights there occasionally. A friend called me one night and said he saw my husband being intimate with another friend of ours. My husband admitted to an affair. It destroyed me, but I also felt sure that I could keep going on my own. My daughters and I moved back to Phoenix and lived for two years with my aunt and her husband. As I examined possible reasons for the breakup, I began to wonder whether I was just less fun, less exciting after our move to Texas. It was something of a blow to my self-confidence as a young woman. Could I be *everything* to someone, or was I lacking some essential "wife" feature?

To have an intimate partnership with someone is to expose ourselves to risk. When we trust someone enough to build a life around our relationship with them, that person becomes a kind of keystone. If our connection to them feels precarious, the entire structure of our lives may feel more precarious, too. That can be a frightening situation. Couples often share not just finances and resources, but children, friends, and important connections to each others' families. Worries about the relationship failing and causing a domino effect on the rest of our lives can be overwhelming, and can seep down into our perception of ourselves. We may wonder, as Aimee did, about our own fitness as a partner, and if we're even capable of fulfilling another person's needs.

If we've been hurt before, and most of us have, we might be reluctant to fully trust an important relationship. Even if we've been with someone for decades, we can still feel a need to protect ourselves.

Mutual, reciprocal vulnerability can lead to stronger and more secure relationships. The ability for partners to trust and be vulnerable with each other—to pause, notice their own and their partner's emotions, and comfortably share their fears—is one of the most powerful relationship skills that a couple can cultivate. It can also relieve a lot of stress, because both partners can get the support they need without having to muster energy in an attempt to be stronger than they really are.

If we do manage to cultivate a strong and trusting bond, we're still not out of the woods, because *even the best relationships are susceptible to decay. Just as trees need water, intimate relationships are living things, and as the seasons of life pass they can't be left to fend for themselves. They need attention, and nourishment.*

THE ENDURING INFLUENCE OF INTIMATE PARTNERSHIPS

Love seems the swiftest, but it is the slowest of all growths. No man or woman really knows what perfect love is until they have been married a quarter of a century.

Mark Twain

Amazing things can happen when a relationship is nurtured over decades. On the other hand, if our most important relationship is neglected, life can devolve into isolation and loneliness.

For illustrations of those two paths, let's go back to Leo DeMarco and John Marsden, two of our First Generation Harvard Study participants. Leo is one of the Study's happiest men, and John one of its unhappiest.

Leo's relationship with his wife, which spanned nearly his entire adult life, contained much of what we've been saying is key to satisfying relationships: affection, curiosity, empathy, and a willingness to face toward challenging emotions and problems, rather than avoid them.

For example, in 1987, Leo's wife, Grace, told the Study that they had some areas of disagreement, including how much time they should spend together, how much sex they should be having, and how often they should be away from home.

When they disagreed, what did they do? They talked about it, she said. They got to know what the other was thinking, and either accepted the difference or worked something out. And just as importantly, they scaffolded this process with affection.

John Marsden's wife, Anne, had different responses to the same questionnaire. She often disagreed with John, she said. But what was most corrosive for their relationship was the lack of affection between them. She believed there should be more—and he also believed there should be more. But they could not figure out how to get there and they didn't talk about it. He rarely confided in her. She rarely confided in him. Were there times, the Study asked, when they were apart and she wished they were together? "Almost never," she said.

The different emotional patterns in each of these marriages stretched through decades of Leo's and John's late lives.

In 2004, we videotaped an interview with Leo in his living room. At one point, the interviewer asks:

"Can you think of five words that describe your relationship with your wife?"

After some stopping and starting, and a few attempts to choose the right words, Leo puts a list together:

Comforting

Challenging

Feisty

Pervasive

Beautiful

Around the same time, in a different part of the country, John Marsden was interviewed in his personal study. In the video he is surrounded by oak shelves full of books, and a bright window to his right looks out on a garden. He's asked the same question—"Can you think of five words that describe your relationship with your wife?"—and he shifts in his chair.

"This is um, this is a required question I suppose?" John asks.

"I wouldn't say it's required," the interviewer responds.

"I'm not sure I could come up with much."

"Just do your best."

John looks around the room and then methodically recites this list:

Tension

Distant

Dismissive

Intolerant

Painful

Most of us have relationships that fall somewhere in between—or even vacillate between—these two extremes. But in these two relationships we see a vivid contrast in the quality of intimacy—a contrast between facing emotional challenges and avoiding them, between affection and distance, between empathy and indifference.

Recall for a moment the Coan handholding study and the Kiecolt-Glaser wound-healing study, which are among the many studies that have shown two crucial findings: First, that the presence of a trusted, intimate partner decreases stress, and second, that stress can affect the healing ability of our bodies. Of course, we can't know exactly how *much* of Leo's and John's late-life health was attributable to the amount of love they felt in their closest relationship, but we do know that Leo was physically active deep into his life, and that John was very ill for many years. Their relationships are not the only reason for that, but the love that Leo shared certainly increased his chances for enduring health, and the pain and distance that John felt in his closest relationship could not have helped him.

The same is true for their wives. Over the course of these couples' lives, their relationships dramatically affected their happiness, life satisfaction, and almost certainly their physical health. It's a story that appears in the Harvard Study again and again.

INTIMACY OVER THE COURSE OF THE LIFESPAN

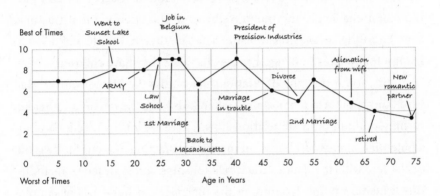

The graph above was made by a First Generation Study participant, Sander Meade, as he looked back on his life when he was in his late 70s. The scale on the left-hand side of the graph represents a rating from the "Best of Times" to the "Worst of Times," and the bottom scale shows a participant's age at the time of each rating. Similar to other participants, many of the big shifts in Sander's life satisfaction coincided with changes in his relationships: age 47: "marriage in trouble"; age 52: "divorce"; age 55: "2nd marriage"; and so on.

Sander's map of his life reflects a key lesson of the Harvard Study and many other research projects: *relationships (and especially intimate relationships) play a crucial role in how satisfied we are at any particular moment in life.*

Life changes of all kinds can cause stress in our intimate partnerships. Even positive changes like getting married can be stressful. Young couples, for example, are often surprised by the relationship challenges that arise when they become parents. What was supposed to be a joyous beginning of family life becomes a minefield of new disagreements and difficulties compounded by exhaustion and worry. New parents often start to have arguments they'd never had before. They are more stressed, and they often feel unsupported by their partners.

This is perfectly normal. Many studies, including our own, show that there is often a decline in relationship satisfaction after the birth of a child; it doesn't mean the relationship is in trouble. Caring for an infant is a major challenge, and much of the time and attention that was once devoted to the couple's relationship must be diverted to the child. So it's natural for couples to struggle somewhat after they have children.

Our careful tracking of relationships across the lifespan in the Harvard Study points to that moment when kids leave the nest as another key turning point in intimate relationships. There are lots of anecdotes about a potential "empty nest boost" in marital satisfaction, but our Study is one of the few with the data to track relationships across decades, including this transition point. Examining the marriages of hundreds of couples, we find that around the time the last child turns 18, partners commonly begin to experience a noticeable increase in relationship satisfaction.

Even Joseph Cichy, who did not have the closest marital relationship, experienced this boost. Using data from the Harvard Study, we can plot lifetime trajectories of marital satisfaction, which often look similar to Joseph's (below). Each vertical dotted line represents the birth of a child, the gray shading represents the time when Joseph and Olivia were raising children under the age of 18, and the dark vertical line represents the year the last child—his daughter Lily—went off to college.

For the men in the Study, this empty nest boost has significance beyond a couple's marital satisfaction. In fact, we found that the *size* of the empty nest boost (it varies across couples) predicted how long these participants would live. The larger the boost in relationship satisfaction after the kids left home, the greater their longevity.

Intimate connections become particularly important in late life. As we age, we encounter more physical challenges, and we need to be able to depend on each other in new ways. When male and female Study

JOSEPH CICHY'S MARITAL SATISFACTION ACROSS TIME

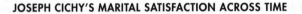

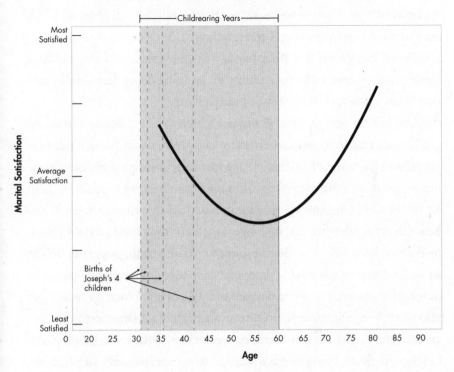

participants were in their late 70s and early 80s, those who were more securely attached to each other reported better mood and fewer disagreements. Two and a half years later, when we checked back in, those securely attached individuals reported feeling more satisfied with life and less depressed, and the wives showed better memory functioning—another piece of evidence suggesting that relationships have an impact on our bodies and brains.

When we look at the spectrum of how individuals in intimate relationships adapted to change and leaned on each other in old age, Leo De-Marco and John Marsden are again at opposite ends. In the interviews we conducted when they were in their 80s, we asked both of them this question:

When you are upset emotionally or sad or worried about something that is not related to your wife, what do you do?

Leo's answer was characteristic of someone who feels the warmth of a secure attachment with a partner: "Go to her. Talk with her," he said. "It's very natural. I certainly don't keep it to myself. She's my confidant."

John's answer, on the other hand, was emblematic of someone who has learned to cope with vulnerability by avoiding dependence on a partner: "I keep it to myself," he said. "I tough it out."

Late life is a time that brings physical challenges and sickness to many. For some of us that means becoming caregivers again (or for the first time), and for some of us that means learning how to accept care. Feeling secure in an intimate relationship means both being available to help a partner and being able to depend on a partner in a time of need. It can be a shock to realize we can no longer reach our own feet to tie our shoes, or that we need help standing up out of a chair. Having a person beside us with whom we are able to share our deepest vulnerabilities can be the difference between a sense of despair and well-being. When we're sick, we also often need someone to act as our advocate—a spokesperson, an organizer, someone to be our hands or eyes or ears . . . or even our memory. On the other side, being that advocate certainly involves self-sacrifice, but it can also be a source of satisfaction.

To put it simply: *couples who are able to face stresses together reap benefits in health, well-being, and relationship satisfaction.*

A FINAL NOTE ABOUT OUR "BETTER HALVES"

In the 1996 romantic comedy *Jerry Maguire*, Tom Cruise famously echoes Plato's notion of love, when he announces to Renée Zellweger, "*You . . . complete me.*"

While the *feeling* that our partners can be our "better halves" still rings true, the practical reality is that very few intimate relationships provide both partners with *everything* they need. Expecting to find completion in our partners can lead to frustration and even the dissolution of otherwise positive relationships.

In his book *The All-or-Nothing Marriage*, psychologist Eli Finkel argues that our expectations of marriage have become unrealistic—particularly in the U.S. and other Western industrialized countries—and that this is part of the reason divorce rates rose sharply in the twentieth century. Before 1850 or so, marriage was essentially a partnership for survival. Between 1850 and 1965, the focus of marriage shifted to include enhanced expectations about companionship and love. In the twenty-first century, a number of factors in the economy and culture have converged in a way that has piled even higher expectations on intimate relationships. People often are less engaged in their local communities, and they relocate more for work. This greater mobility means that fewer people are living near extended family. Many do not stay in one place long enough to build stable groups of friends. Who do we expect to fill all of these gaps? The person beside us.

Without realizing it, many of us expect our partners to provide money, love, sex, and to be our best friends. We expect them to provide counsel and conversation and to make us laugh. We want them to help us become our best selves. We not only ask our partners to do these things for us; we also expect to provide these things for them. A lucky few may find themselves in relationships where these high expectations are met reasonably well. In most relationships, it's too much to ask.

How do our close relationships get weighted down with so much expectation? Sometimes the reason has less to do with the relationship and more to do with waning connections in other parts of our lives. If we're no longer having the kind of fun we can only have with a group of friends or family members who know us well, or we've stopped pursuing our personal interests, hobbies, and passions, we might turn to our partner to fill those needs. The intimate relationship becomes like a sponge, soaking up whatever failed expectation happens to be lying around. Suddenly we're finding fault with the person beside us when it's the rest of our lives and our other relationships that need attention. These expectations can take a toll.

The research is clear: intimate relationships can be an incredible source of sustenance for our minds and bodies. But there are limits to what they can do. If we want to give a relationship the best chance of success, we have to support it by sustaining other parts of our lives. Our partners may in fact be our better halves, but they can't, by themselves, make us whole.

THE PATH AHEAD

> There is no remedy for love but to love more.
>
> Henry David Thoreau

As you think about how the things we've discussed in this chapter map onto your own life, consider using the following practices to nudge a relationship in the direction you'd like it to go.

"Catch" your partner being kind. What was the last thing your partner did that you felt grateful for? A dinner he made? A backrub she gave you? Or maybe there was a moment you were impatient with your partner, but he didn't hold it against you, and you appreciated that.

Take note of that small act. Research points to the benefits of keeping a gratitude diary to record and solidify the things we feel grateful for, but even simply noticing and calling to mind the good, little things your partner does can have a positive impact. This is a simple but powerful way for us to "catch" our partners being kind rather than falling into the common trap of giving more attention to disappointments. Expressing our gratitude to our partner increases the impact further. There are reasons we connected to our partners in the first place, and reasons they make our lives better now—it's good to remember those reasons (and to mention them!). It feels good to be appreciated.

Step out of old routines. As we go about the business of life, our relationships can begin to feel like they are stuck in repetitive cycles that are not exciting.

Every night: dinner and TV.

Every morning: coffee and oatmeal.

Every Sunday: mow the lawn, go to the grocery store, cook the same dinner.

Try something different! Make a plan to surprise your partner with breakfast in bed. Maybe you haven't walked around your neighborhood together in years—after dinner instead of falling into the grooves of your usual routine, take a stroll and see what's out there. Plan a weekly date night and take turns choosing what you will do (and maybe surprise your partner with a new activity if a surprise would be welcome).

We all fall into habits and routines. That's normal. But often they become so rote that we cease to really notice our partners as we cruise through the day. Breaking these routines alerts our minds to novelty, and this helps us recognize and appreciate our partners in new ways. It also signals to our partners that they are important to us.

And there's always dance class . . .

Try the W.I.S.E.R. model (squared). When disagreements arise, consider using the W.I.S.E.R. model (from Chapter Six), and sharing the techniques with your partner. The *watch* and *interpret* steps are especially useful in intimate relationships. Taking extra time to watch ourselves and our partners in an emotional situation can help us see with greater clarity the reasons behind the emotions we are feeling. Introducing some stillness into a moment of turmoil can help us clear the muddy water below the surface of our relationship.

So when you bump up against something about your partner that bothers you, before reacting, pause to *watch*, and take note of your reactions and what you are thinking.

Then *interpret* your feelings and try to make sense of what's going on. Ask: *Why is this issue important to me? What exactly is my view? Where does it come from? Is this something I learned from my family growing up? Something I learned from previous relationships? Something that was emphasized in my religious training?*

Then, the harder part: try to step into your partner's shoes. *Why is my partner having such a strong reaction, behaving in this particular way, thinking this particular thing? Why might it be important to my partner and where might my partner have learned this? Where is it coming from?*

Sometimes it's difficult to start conversations about challenging topics, and difficult to move interactions in a new direction. The waters of old grievances tend to run deep. Just telling your partner that the topic makes you anxious is a good start. There are a few additional techniques that might be useful in that case.

One is known as "reflective listening." It helps us make sure we're hearing correctly what our partner is trying to say, and it shows that we care, that we are trying to empathize. It works like this:

First, listen *without commenting*.

Then, try to communicate what you've heard your partner say *without judgment* (this is the hard part). You might begin with something like: *What I'm hearing you say is ___. Is that right?*

A second technique that is helpful in its own right and can make reflective listening even more valuable is to offer some understanding of your partner's reasons for a feeling or behavior. The goal is not to point out your brilliance and ability to see things your partner cannot, but to let your partner know that you see them. You want to communicate that it makes sense that she feels this way or that he is behaving in that way, and to nurture that bedrock of empathy and affection that research has shown to be valuable. For example, you might say, *It makes sense that you feel so strongly about this* . . . and then continue with something like: *since you care so much about being kind.* Or: *. . . since this was the way you've described things happening in your family growing up.*

A third useful practice is to try to step back a bit from the conversation, a practice that psychologists call "self-distancing," and look at your experience as if you are watching someone else. You might notice the thoughts that this person (i.e., you) is having, and recognize them as fleeting thoughts that may shift. This is a technique that shares much in common with mindfulness approaches, and the psychologists Ethan Kross and Ozlem Ayduk have done a lot of research showing its utility.

Together these practices may help you to get started with challenging conversations and hang in there emotionally when things get tough, to slow down, and to show your partner that you're trying to understand.

Don't be afraid to come up with some of your own practices that work in your particular relationship. When you feel yourself getting angry or feeling defeated or scared, remember that it's a signal. Reach out to your partner in those moments. Try to see beneath the surface, and remember that just like you, your partner is also fighting battles.

We each bring our own particular strengths and weaknesses into a relationship, our own fears and desires, enthusiasms and anxieties, and the dance that results will always be unlike any other.

"We don't harbor resentment," Grace DeMarco told the Study in 2004, referring to her relationship with Leo. "When we're pushed hard enough, we really say what we feel, get it out in the open. You can be very different but still respect that difference. And we *need* the difference, actually. He needs the lightening up and I need the settling down."

8

FAMILY MATTERS

Call it a clan, call it a network, call it a tribe, call it a family: Whatever you call it, whoever you are, you need one.

Jane Howard, author

Harvard Study Questionnaire, 1990

```
Q: When you think about your family and relatives, with
about how many of them do you think you would say:

    We share most of our joys and sorrows _____
    We enjoy doing things together; we share interests
    _____
    We really don't make an effort to keep up with one
    another _____
    We avoid each other or we probably don't like each other
    much _____
```

Reading through any file in the Harvard Study can feel a lot like looking through a family photo album, or watching a montage of old 8mm film. Many of the records are handwritten in cursive, the stories themselves are steeped in the diction and the feeling of past eras, and time seems to move incredibly fast. Entire generations of families go by with the flick of a few pages. A participant is born, speeds through his teens, gets married, and suddenly a boy who was only 14 years old moments ago is now 85, and his adult children are in our offices talking about what he was like as a parent. Although there are many insights that have come from the close inspection of detailed data from the Study, a casual look through any file quickly puts two particular things into perspective: 1) the pace at which human life unfolds, and 2) the significance of family.

"We had a big family, and I'm grateful for the experience of that," one of our Second Generation participants, Linda, told the Study in 2018 when she visited our offices in the West End of Boston. Her father was Neal "Mac" McCarthy, one of the Study's most dedicated First Generation participants, and he'd grown up on Lowell Street (now Lomasney Way), not far from where she now sat. "There was a lot of energy in our family, a lot of love," Linda told us. "But when I think of my dad I get emotional because he came from a totally different situation. He had some hard times as a kid and his family broke apart. He didn't finish high school. Went to war. Came out of all of that and got his feet under him and somehow he was still a great dad, always there for us, always loving. His life could have gone a completely different direction. I have a lot of respect for him."

No relationships are quite like the ones we have with our families. For better or worse, our family members are often the people most involved in our lives when we're young and developing, and who know us for the longest stretch of time. Our parents are the first human beings we see when we arrive in the world, the first people to hold and nurture us, and much of what we learn to expect from close relationships comes from them. Our siblings, if we have them, are among our first contemporaries, who show us how to behave and also how to get into trouble. Our extended family often defines how we understand the meaning of community. But whatever the makeup of our family, it is more than a group of relationships; it is, in a very real way, part of who we are. So these relationships come with some very high stakes. Their character can have a dramatic effect on our well-being.

But the nature and size of this effect is an ongoing debate in the field of psychology. Some believe that early family experience determines who we become. Others think its effect is largely overrated, and that genes are more important. Because every one of us has had a long history of first-hand experience with our own families, each of us tends to have strong opinions about how families work, and how much they affect or determine our lives. From that personal experience come important assumptions about what is and is not possible (both in our families of origin and the new families that we create) and these assumptions often determine how we conduct those relationships.

We sometimes think, for example, that the way our family is now is the way it will always be, that those relationships are set in stone. We also tend to paint both our early and current family experiences in absolute, black-and-white terms: *My parents were horrible . . . My childhood was idyllic . . . My family was clueless . . . My in-laws are intrusive . . . My daughter's an angel . . .* Are family connections really as frozen across time as we often picture them?

The Harvard Study captures an enormous range of family experience over many decades, and it can help to shed some light on how families really work over time. Close bonds, family feuds, and all variety of successes and struggles are represented. We have the accounts of relationships between parents and children as seen from both sides. We have "traditional" nuclear family households, single-parent households, multigenerational households, families with adopted children, families blended through divorce and remarriage, and families with siblings who function more like parents. On top of all of that, more than 40 percent of participants had at least one parent who'd immigrated to the U.S. from another country and faced the challenges of raising a family in a foreign land.

Neal McCarthy's family was one of these. As first-generation Irish immigrants, his mother and father arrived in the United States only months before Neal was born, and had their fair share of troubles trying to integrate into a new society. As we'll see, Neal's childhood had both nurturing and traumatic elements, and his daughter Linda was right—his life could have easily gone in a more negative direction. Many lives in the Harvard Study did. But Neal managed to come out ahead and to live a full and vibrant life that included a loving family of his own. His path through life is both moving and instructive.

In 2012, when he was 84, Neal mailed in our biennial questionnaire and on the back wrote a note to Robin Western, one of the Study's long-term coordinators. The note suggests the flavor of his life at the time, and how far he'd come from his early struggles in Boston's West End:

Dear Robin,

Trust this finds you well along with your family.

Can't believe I've been in this Study for over 70 years!

Although I'm now 84, I'm still very active with my family and friends. Babysitting my five-year-old granddaughter keeps grandpa Mac on his toes, also holiday get-togethers are always fun! I read books, do crossword puzzles and attend my 7 grandchildren's school and sports activities.

Wishing your family and you the best always.

Would love to hear from you and get an update since we last met.

Best always,
Neal McCarthy (Mac)

If we'd shown this joyful note to Neal when he was 16 and living through the depths of his family struggles, he might have been very surprised. He traveled a long, long way in his life, and faced some extremely difficult choices along the way. Indeed, one common theme among all of the Harvard Study families, regardless of the size or closeness of the family, the joys or the challenges, is the steady march of change.

At any one moment a single family can reflect the entire human life cycle—with infants, adolescents, and adults at every stage of life all in relationship to each other. As the life cycle continues to turn, every family member finds themselves on new perches, playing new roles. These shifting roles always require some adaptation. Parents who only recently were giving their adolescent child rides to parties and helping with homework soon have to learn to respect her growing independence as she transitions into adulthood. Siblings have to negotiate changes in their relationship dynamics as their life paths diverge. Adult children have to come to terms with providing support to their aging parents and eventually, in one of the more difficult role changes, to accept late-life support themselves. These transitions require more than adaptation to new roles and responsibilities; they require emotional adaptation, too.

As time passes, and everyone's life stage shifts, relationships must change. *How a family adapts to that inevitable change is one of the key determinants of the quality of family relationships.* We can't forever remain the small child with ever-watchful parents, or the young adult in the first swells of romantic love, or the new retiree with a grandchild giggling on his or her knee. It doesn't matter how tightly we hang on to a particular beloved perch in life; eventually that perch begins to crumble. We have to keep moving, facing into new roles and novel challenges, and it's always easier to do that together. But how?

The emotional lattice of every family is as unique as the structure of a flower; similar to other families on first glance, but one of a kind upon close inspection. For some of us our family evokes a sense of warm belonging, for some a feeling of estrangement, or even fear. For most of us . . . it's complicated. This complexity makes research challenging, but by closely following hundreds of families over many decades, the Harvard Study is in a unique position to find points of overlap among families, and to discover some of the common factors that define the character of our family relationships. This chapter is about bringing together critical pieces of this research to create a different kind of lens through which you can view the particularity of your own family life. Because one of the resounding truths that we find in the Harvard Study over and over is this: family matters.

WHAT IS A FAMILY?

No man is an island
Entire of itself,
Every man is a piece of the continent,
A part of the main.

John Donne

It can be tempting to believe that each of us has more control over our own fate than we actually do. The truth is that we are all embedded in ecologies bigger than ourselves that shape us in profound ways. Economies, cultures, and subcultures all play important roles in what we believe, how we behave, and the progression of our lives. None of these ecologies is more important than that of the family.

But what is a family, exactly? For most of us, when we think of family, we think of *our* family. But while for one person family might consist of biological parents, siblings, and children, for another it might mean step-relationships or an enormous range of extended family—in-laws, cousins, second cousins, nieces and nephews. For others it might extend even further, to important connections that go beyond blood relation.

Any definition of "family" begins with the culture that surrounds it. In ancient China, the idea of family was shaped by Confucianism and a collectivist ideology that emphasized the health and success of the entire group. A single household would include parents, grandparents, and children, and be the center of life. This model remains strong in China today, even in the era of one-child families. In Ancient Rome a family consisted of all members of a household, including workers and servants, who lived under the rule of the oldest male, the *pater familias*. In modern Western culture, the "nuclear family," consisting of two parents and their children, is a common definition of family, despite the numerous alternatives to this prototype.

"I have five mommies but only one daddy," one participant told the Study when he was 14. His adoptive parents already had grandchildren when he joined their family, and he considered his adoptive mother, her two sisters, and her two biological daughters to all be mother figures.

A family can consist of many different arrangements and levels of closeness or distance. Those who haven't felt the warmth and presence of family members, whose families have been abusive or have failed to understand them, may long for and find other connections that feel family-like and provide many of the things that they need. One person might have no relationship with their father, but be very close to an uncle, or a grandparent, or a different adult from their childhood, like a soccer coach or the mother of a close friend. Or they might find family in an entirely different community altogether.

In New York City, Detroit, and many other urban areas in the U.S., a rich example of nontraditional family can be found in "Ballroom culture," in which members of the LGBTQ+ community, most of them Black and Latino, join groups known as "houses" and organize their lives around supporting one another and competing together in drag ballroom competitions. Houses provide much needed, family-like connections around shared experiences, goals, and values. Every house functions in a similar way to a blood family, with a house "mother" or "father" who takes on many of the roles of a traditional parent, and provides some of the positive structure and connection many of the house's "children" may have missed out on earlier in their lives.

As Marlon M. Bailey puts it in his 2013 book about Ballroom culture, *Butch Queens Up in Pumps* (whose title identifies the ballroom category that Bailey himself competed in): "In general, a 'house' does not signify an actual building; rather it represents the ways in which its members, who mostly live in various locations, view themselves and interact with each other as a family unit. . . . Indeed, especially for LGBTQ+ people of color in their late teens and early twenties, this community offers an enduring social sanctuary for those who have been rejected by and marginalized within their families of origin, religious institutions, and society at large."

The essential point is that close, nurturing units of people that have a formative effect on our lives can come from a variety of places, include a variety of people, and be called any number of things. *What matters is not just who we consider to be family, but what our closest relationships mean to us over the course of our lives.*

This doesn't diminish the importance of families of origin, however. Even when new families form, or we become a part of new communities that provide us a family structure, we all still carry with us the history of our families of origin and the experiences that have impacted us, both positive and negative. Even created families, in all of their beauty, and with all of their love, exist in relief against that earlier experience. Regardless of our current lives, we still carry the ghosts of our childhoods, and our memories of the people who raised us.

THE GHOSTS OF CHILDHOOD

At the back of a drawer in Bob's kitchen is an old aluminum ice cream scoop that belonged to his mother. When he was a kid, he'd come in after running around his Des Moines neighborhood on a summer day and she'd use that scoop to dish up some ice cream for him and maybe have a little bit herself. Now more than sixty years later he pulls out that scoop and it's a little bit like pulling a memory out of a drawer. The smell of his mother's kitchen, the feeling of that moment in time, is somehow embedded in the ice cream scoop.

Marc has similar heirlooms. On his desk he keeps a small plaque with his grandfather's name on it. His grandfather was a builder, and displayed the plaque on his own desk. When Marc looks at it, he remembers his grandfather teaching him how to use a hammer and nail. He can almost hear the sound of his grandfather's voice, simultaneously gruff and kind.

Many of us tend to keep items of significance from our family that represent things that have meaning for us—both good and bad. Certain objects can connect us evocatively to the way things used to be, remind us of how far we've come and of lessons we've learned.

These heirlooms are tokens of a larger kind of inheritance. Not just of objects, but of perspectives, habits, philosophies, and experiences. We can hold on to psychological heirlooms just as surely as we hold on to something like an ice scream scoop. Bob's mother always emphasized being purposely kind as a way to connect with others—waiters, strangers, anyone—and today Bob finds himself trying to follow suit. Marc's grandfather used to talk often about the pleasure of doing things well, how there's a certain sound when a hammer strikes a nail just right, and though Marc's not building houses, he thinks of that simple lesson often.

There is also a darker side of these inheritances, the difficult, even traumatic experiences of childhood that make imprints on us psychologically. Marc's father's experience of *Kristallnacht* and escaping the Holocaust remained with him for life. Many Harvard Study participants struggled with bullying or abusive parents.

Psychological inheritances can run very deep—sometimes too deep to easily recognize. Beyond the physical features that we inherit from our biological parents, we acquire habits, perspectives, and models of behavior from family members. Our most important experiences, both good and bad, are not just memories. They are emotional events that leave tangible impressions on us, and these influences can shape our lives for a very long time.

This can be true for any experience, at any stage of life, but it's especially relevant for the experiences a child has within their family of origin. There's been a great deal of research and writing about the importance of childhood experience, leading to a wide variety of common assumptions about the role childhood plays in adult life. In popular culture, movies, and media, a person's difficult childhood is often cited as the reason they've behaved a certain way, so much so that it seems like an accepted truism that childhood determines one's fate in life. In a television show, when we are given the backstory of a murderous villain, it always seems to be that they were abused as a child. The trope is so pervasive that those of us who've had a rough time as a kid often worry: *If I had a terrible childhood am I somehow irreparably broken? Am I doomed to an unhappy life?*

TROUBLE IN PARADISE

In 1955, a developmental psychologist named Emmy Werner was trying to better understand the significance of difficult childhood experiences, so she started a longitudinal study on the Hawaiian island of Kauai designed to follow children from the very day they were born all the way into their adulthood. Many of the families she studied were struggling in much the same way as immigrant families living in Boston when the Harvard Study began. As Werner wrote:

[The participants] were children and grandchildren of immigrants from Southeast Asia and Europe, who had come to Hawaii to work on the sugar plantations. About half came from families in which the fathers were semiskilled or unskilled laborers and the mothers had less than eight years of education. . . . [They were] Japanese, Filipino, Hawaiians, and part-Hawaiians, Portuguese, Puerto-Ricans, Chinese, Koreans, and a small group of Anglo-Saxon Caucasians.

What made this study so remarkable is that Werner didn't select just a few participants from the island; she managed to include every child born on the island of Kauai in 1955—690 total—and the study lasted for over thirty years.

Using data from their childhoods, adolescence, and adult lives, Werner was able to show a clear connection between adverse childhood events and the trajectory of well-being in individual lives. Those children who had a complicated illness at birth, who had poor experiences with their caretakers, and who suffered abuse were more likely to have mental health problems and to develop learning disabilities. Their childhood experience really mattered.

But Werner also found reasons for hope.

One third of all children who had adverse childhoods still managed to develop into attentive, kind, and emotionally well-adjusted adults. These kids overcame their difficult childhoods, and Werner was able to point to some of the reasons.

There were protective factors at work for some children that countered the effects of their difficult childhoods. One of the major sources of protection was the consistent presence of at least one caring adult. Even one person who is concerned, available, and emotionally invested in a child's well-being can positively affect that child's development and future relationships. Some of the children who thrived despite adversity seemed particularly able to elicit this kind of caring support.

As adults, the Harvard Study participants who were able to acknowledge challenges and talk about them more openly seemed to have a similar ability to elicit support from others. Being open and clear about one's experiences offers an opportunity for another person to be helpful. This ability to acknowledge and deal with rather than try to ignore challenges may play an important role in eliciting support both in childhood and later. Neal McCarthy's life is a wonderful illustration of how this works, and how we might build on our family experiences—good and bad—in a way that helps us thrive.

THE ORIGINS (AND DEVELOPMENT) OF OUR COPING ABILITIES

On a cold Saturday afternoon in November of 1942, a Harvard Study interviewer visited Neal McCarthy's family for the first time at their home in Boston's West End. If we flip to the very beginning of Neal's records, we can find the interviewer's notes from that day. Their three-room apartment was lively and bustling, the interviewer wrote, with the six kids doing chores and joking around, saying hello to the stranger in a shirt and tie sitting at their kitchen table. One of Neal's brothers was washing the dishes that had piled up. Neal was busy teaching his youngest sister how to tie her shoes. He was 14 years old.

In the late 1930s and early 1940s, researchers conducted these visits to the homes of our First Generation participants to see what their family lives were like. How strict and how kind were their parents? How present? How involved? Did the parents have a consistent positive emotional connection with their children, or were they withdrawn or only sporadically attentive? Did the family argue a lot? In short: How warm and supportive were these children's family environments?

Both Neal's parents were born in Ireland and immigrated to the U.S. only months before Neal was born. During the Study's first visit, Mary, Neal's mother, made tea for the interviewer and sat at the kitchen table answering questions about the family's history. Occasionally one of the kids would come through to announce the completion of a task or ask permission to go see a friend. "The children all respect Neal's mother," the interviewer wrote. "She is a kind and good-natured person and the children do center around her and there is a warm affection both ways. She is particularly proud of Neal because he is so good and she doesn't have to worry about him."

Like many of the participants in the inner-city sample, Neal worked from a very young age. He started delivering groceries and newspapers at age 10, and on Sundays he'd go into the wealthy "lace curtain Irish neighborhood" across town and shine shoes for people as they were coming out of church. Remembering these early years as an older man, Neal told the Study that he gave most of the money he made to his mother to use for family expenses. "I'd bring my take home and give her usually about four bucks. And she'd think that was pretty good. But she wouldn't know I had a buck in my hat!" Many afternoons he'd go to the bowling alley and set up pins so they'd let him play for free.

His mother paid special attention to who Neal chose as friends, and when the interviewer asked Neal why he thought he had stayed out of trouble in a neighborhood where many of his peers had not, Neal said, "I don't run around with dumbbells."

Neal's father, a dockworker, was also well respected by the children. He was kind and firm, though it was clear that his mother ran the household.

Neal was one of a large sample of Harvard Study participants that we used to investigate the effect of childhood experience on participants' adult lives. We wanted to know: Could the echo of early family experiences be heard throughout a person's entire life? With careful notes and ratings from initial visits like the one to Neal's family home, we were able to form pictures of participants' childhood family environments. In Neal's case, the family environment was considered very positive. His parents were nurturing, involved, consistent, and fostered their children's autonomy. The family environment as a whole was rated as warm and cohesive.

Now let's flip forward in the record to more than sixty years later, when we interviewed participants in their homes when they were in their 70s and 80s. During these visits we paid particular attention to the security of their connections with their partners. Did they display loving behavior? Were they comfortable in seeking and giving support? Did they value or devalue their partner? We relied not just on the face value of their responses but also the believability and consistency of their comments.

When we interviewed Neal and his wife, Gail, it quickly became clear that they were securely attached. When asked separately to describe their relationship, the words they chose were remarkably similar. *Loving, communicative, tender, affectionate, comfortable*, Neal said. *Tender, open, giving, understanding, affectionate*, Gail said. And they both provided rich examples in their interviews to support these adjectives in a persuasive way. At that time, Gail was becoming increasingly incapacitated by Parkinson's disease, and had been struggling with it for several years. They were living in Seattle, Washington, where Neal ran an accounting firm that he cofounded, and Gail talked about how Neal had changed his professional life to help care for her, taking on only as many clients as he could handle while still giving her the necessary attention. He learned to cook her favorite meals and took over all the household responsibilities. But she insisted that he keep up his hobby of birdwatching, saying "Find a good one for me!" on his way out the door.

"I've learned a lot about warblers," she told the Study.

This research in a way bookended the lives of our participants. We purposely went to the far extremes of the data—the very beginning and close to the end—looking for associations between childhood and late-life functioning. Given the passage of over six decades, we ourselves were not certain this kind of connection across relationships would be found. But our hypothesis proved accurate: the men who, like Neal, had closer and warmer experiences in early family life were more likely to be able to connect with, depend on, and support their partner more than sixty years later. The strength of the connection across sixty years was not immense, but it was clear that our participants' childhoods were like long, thin threads, gently tugging on their adult lives from across the decades.

After discovering this link came the crucial question: How does this work? How exactly does the quality of people's childhoods affect their adult lives?

Here is where Emmy Werner's research, our own Harvard Study research, and many other pieces of research from across cultures and populations converge to show that *a critical link between childhood experience and positive adult social connections is our ability to process emotions.*

It is from our relationships as children—especially our relationships with our family—that we first learn what to expect from others. This is when we begin to develop the emotional habits, so to speak, that will be with us for the rest of our lives. These habits often define the way we connect to others and our ability to engage others in mutually supportive ways.

A crucial point here is that *our ability to process emotions is malleable. In fact, managing emotions is one of the things we actually get better at as we grow old. And there is strong evidence that we don't have to wait until late in our lives for this to happen. With the right guidance and some practice, we can learn to be better at managing our feelings at any age.*

The connections between our childhood experience and our adult lives are not so strong that they can't be altered. Any experience we have, even as adults, has the power to change us. There are participants in the Study, for example, who had warm and loving childhoods, but then had difficult experiences later on that changed the way they approached relationships. There are also participants who had difficult childhoods, but their later experiences helped them learn how to trust and connect with others.

Neal is a particularly interesting and encouraging case for exactly this reason, because while his early childhood was about as positive an experience as can be found in the Harvard Study, that warmth did not last forever. Shortly after the Harvard Study's first visit, everything changed for the McCarthy family, and the coming years would put the positive habits he'd learned as a child to the test.

TROUBLE IN THE MCCARTHY FAMILY

When the Harvard Study first visited Neal's family, his mother was extremely candid about many details of their family life, painting a broad and realistic picture of the family's ups and downs. But there was one crucial thing she did not mention during that first visit: she had personally begun struggling, mightily, with an addiction to alcohol.

For many years Mary had managed her drinking in ways that did not interfere with raising the children and keeping her family thriving. She drank in private, and managed to control the amount and timing of her drinking. But shortly after the Study's first visit to the McCarthy home, Mary began to lose control. Soon she was drinking to intoxication every day. The household became tumultuous and even traumatic for the children as she and Neal's father began to have loud, raucous fights about her drinking and the way it was affecting the family. There would be screaming and sometimes violence, from both Neal's parents. Neal loved his parents, and in an effort to support his fracturing family, he dropped out of high school at 15 to go to work. He lived at home until he was 19, helping to support the family and provide a stable resource for his younger siblings. As we've seen in previous cases, his experience of taking on early work and responsibility was not unusual for the inner-city Study participants.

Neal carried vivid memories of this period of turmoil with him for the rest of his life—the shouting, the violence and injuries, the stress, his mother's drunkenness and the family's pervading sadness. He lived at home until he felt like he could no longer do anything more to help.

"I just had to leave," he told a Study interviewer, tearfully, when he was in his 60s. "I had to. My mother was an alcoholic. Her and Daddy used to fight."

Like many of the children in Werner's Kauai longitudinal study, Neal's family life was a complex, unfolding web of experience and feeling, of love and frustration, of closeness and estrangement, of good and bad. Neal's family, like most families, was complicated.

But Neal's case shows the power that we all have to define our own story. He experienced first a warm, loving childhood environment, and later—when his mother descended into alcoholism—a tumultuous and difficult adolescence. Both experiences affected him deeply. Yet he was able to draw on his positive experiences in order to put his negative experiences in perspective, rather than the other way around. He also had that one present, attentive adult in his life—his dad. Together, these resources gave him the strength and confidence to handle any emotional challenge he faced.

"I knew that wasn't how I wanted to live," he told the Study about his teenage years, and watching his parents. "Fighting, drinking, screaming. When I got older I didn't want my kids experiencing that, and I didn't want to experience it myself, ever again."

At the age of 19, Neal escaped his family home by enlisting in the Army. He fought in the Korean War, and when he was discharged he got his high school GED. He used his veterans benefits to go to college, where he met Gail, and fell in love. Exactly eleven days after he graduated college, Neal and Gail were married. Only a short time later his mother died of complications related to her drinking. She was only 55.

Over a lifetime of experience, Neal developed his ability to reflect on whatever might happen to him and to consider his own emotions before acting. He was able to step back, acknowledge his challenges, and give himself the space to find a path forward. And he would need these skills. Neal might have had a tumultuous, traumatic adolescence, and fought in a war, but according to him, it wasn't until he'd had a family and children of his own that he faced the most difficult challenge of his life.

NEAL MEETS THE UNEXPECTED CHALLENGES OF FAMILY LIFE

By the time he was 56, Neal "Mac" McCarthy and his wife, Gail, were the proud parents of four children, all adults. Each of his kids, he told the Study, was smarter than he was and—he emphasized—kind. His oldest son and daughter, twins, had both gone to college. His son was now an accountant and his daughter Linda (the Second Generation participant we heard from at the beginning of this chapter) got her PhD and became a chemist. This achievement amazed Neal; Linda was the first PhD in his family. His middle son married young and was living in Costa Rica. His youngest daughter, Lucy, was a brilliant kid, he said, with a lot of potential. As an adolescent, Lucy was fascinated by astrophysics and space, and dreamed of becoming an engineer for NASA. "She's so smart it's scary," Neal said at the time.

But as the years went by certain challenges arose for Lucy that neither Neal nor Gail knew how to handle. Lucy had been shy, had a hard time making friends as a child, and was bullied in primary school. Her home life was a safe haven, and her brothers and sister looked out for her, but her experience away from home continued to be a challenge. In high school, she made few new friends, began skipping classes, and, unbeknownst to her parents for several years, started drinking to excess. After high school Lucy continued to live with Neal and Gail. She was fired from several jobs for absences and would sometimes spend days in her room, not wanting to come out. Once she was arrested for stealing a watch from a department store.

Lucy's drinking was especially alarming to Neal because of his mother's experience. Had he passed on some addiction genes to Lucy? Would she follow in his mother's footsteps?

The family rallied around Lucy as best they could. Her siblings were available to her, and her older brother Tim called her often to check in. Lucy felt more comfortable talking to him about some things, and felt more comfortable talking to her parents about other things. Neal and Gail gave her the space she seemed to prefer, but they didn't want to detach too much. Gail made an effort to find the right therapist for her—going through several before finding one that Lucy was at ease with. Often Lucy would seem to be improving, only to fall on hard times again. She was diagnosed with depression and began taking medication. That helped, but it wasn't a complete solution. Lucy's two oldest siblings had gone to college, and she wanted to do the same, but when it came time to apply, she couldn't bring herself to do it. She started working at restaurants around Seattle instead, living with her parents and sometimes trying to venture out and live by herself. Once, when Lucy was 25, Neal came home from work between meetings to find her at the kitchen table, sobbing uncontrollably, saying she didn't want to live anymore. He didn't know what to say to her, and was afraid of saying the wrong thing. He canceled his appointments and made coffee and sandwiches and sat with her. She left crying before her mother could come home.

"We don't know what to do," Neal told the Study. "We try to be there for her but we feel like we're out of options. I make sure to tell her I love her. She's living on her own now and I lend her resources when she needs them. She never wants to take money but sometimes I have to insist because I don't want to see her living on the street. Ever since she was a kid I've given probably 80 percent of my attention to Lucy because of her troubles, and the other kids got the last 20 percent. They never complained but I know it was hard for them. That's just the way it is, I guess."

Lucy's problems complicated her transition into adulthood, but her situation contained the same developmental dilemmas that all families face with young adults: when should a parent intervene rather than step back, and what kind of support is best? From the young adult's side the same dilemma exists in mirror image: How do I get what I need from my parents when things are not going well, yet still work toward being as grown-up as I think I should be?

Every family faces challenges, and sometimes these problems are not really fixable. There is a Western idea, particularly in the United States, that we ought to be able to conquer all problems. If a problem doesn't seem conquerable, the response is often to turn away entirely. The choices become: *I must do everything*, or *I can't do anything*.

But there is a middle way. We've been advocating a strategy of facing toward problems, rather than avoiding them, but *facing* a problem is not always the same as *fixing* it. Sometimes facing-in to our families means learning how to sit with uncomfortable situations and emotions, and allowing ourselves to feel and express the emotions that many of us try to avoid. Sometimes the best thing we can do is respond in a way that is less absolute and more flexible, as Neal and Gail managed to do.

Neal and Gail were at a crossroad: Should they try their best to engage with Lucy and her challenges? Or should they back off a bit and give Lucy more room to either flounder or thrive on her own? While they struggled with these questions, their response was most often to face toward Lucy's difficulty rather than minimizing it or pretending there was not a problem. When Lucy pushed them away, they didn't throw their hands up and cut her off. Instead, they gave her room, and waited for another opportunity. Lucy's siblings also gave needed support to their parents and to Lucy. All through the experience, even in times of shouting and fighting, the family's love for each other would eventually surface. They remained flexible, though none of them was perfect. Sometimes they had to step back, sometimes they had to step in. But *they never turned away*.

Still, like many in his situation, Neal couldn't help but wonder if any of this was the right strategy. It was hard to tell if they were doing the right things, and he worried about his own contributions to Lucy's misery.

"Can I get your professional opinion?" Neal once asked a Study interviewer, thirty years his junior, in a discussion about his daughter. "Is there anything more I can do for her? Do you think I've done something wrong?"

It's natural to feel responsible for our kids' failures as well as their successes, even when much of it is not within our control. Parents often face feelings of guilt when their children encounter problems in life.

Sometimes these guilty feelings become yet another reason to turn away from problems; we just can't handle facing those emotions. It took bravery on Neal's part to give voice to a question that many parents find themselves asking when their children have difficulties in life: *Is it my fault?*

Neal never managed to answer this question fully for himself; it stayed on his mind even as Lucy aged into her 30s and 40s still experiencing ups and downs, periods of homelessness, and problems with addiction.

It's true that childhood matters, and parenting matters, but no single element of a person's life fully shapes their future. Parents can neither take as much credit nor as much blame as they think they should for the way their children turn out. Nature and nurture, heredity and environment, parenting and peers are all tightly woven together, and all have served to mold each of us into the adults we are today. Finding a definitive reason for why a particular person is having the struggles they are having is not always possible. All we can do is to meet our emotions, as Neal did, with as much bravery as we can, and respond in the best way we know how.

CORRECTIVE EXPERIENCES (AND STARTING NOW)

So what do we do if most of our childhood experience was incredibly rough, or even traumatic? Is there still hope for those of us who, unlike Neal, had nothing but trouble when we were young?

The answer is an emphatic *Yes*. There is hope. This goes for everyone, whether your experience in childhood was difficult, or whether you find yourselves having troubles today. Childhood isn't the only time of life when experience is formative. Anything we experience, at any time, can change what we expect from others. It often happens that a powerful, positive experience will have a corrective effect on an earlier, negative experience. If we grew up with a domineering father, we might later become close with a friend whose father behaves in a completely different way. Because the friend's father doesn't live up to our worst expectations, our perspective can undergo a subtle shift. Now we might be more open to other possibilities.

We are having these experiences all the time, whether we realize it or not. Life, in a way, is a long opportunity for corrective experiences. Finding the right partner, for example, can go a long way toward correcting assumptions and expectations that we developed in childhood. Therapy can also be helpful, in part because of the connection with a caring, consistent adult.

Corrective experiences aren't just a matter of luck, either. Opportunities to shift our view of the world are arriving all the time—most of them simply pass us by. We are often too tunneled into our own expectations and personal opinions to allow the subtle realities of these opportunities to penetrate. But there are a couple of simple (though difficult!) things we can do to encourage our ability to see what's really happening, and thus be more likely to reap the benefits of corrective experience.

First, we can tune in to difficult feelings rather than try to ignore them. Part of leaning in to challenges involves seeing our emotional reactions as useful information rather than as something to be pushed away.

Second, we can notice when we are having experiences that are more positive than we expected. Maybe in the middle of that family reunion you were dreading for months, you can pause and realize that, against all odds, you're having a pretty good time.

Third, we can try to "catch" other people when they are behaving well, just as we suggested you might do with a partner. Most of us are very good at noticing when people are behaving badly, but we're not so skilled at noticing when people are behaving well. On the road, good drivers fade into the background, but bad drivers stand out. We learn to expect bad driving, so that we're prepared for it when it happens. The same is true in life. Occasionally, try to notice the good drivers, the good people.

The final and most powerful approach is simply to remain open to the possibility of people behaving differently than we expect. *The more ready we are to be surprised by people, the more likely we are to notice when they do something that doesn't match our expectation.* This kind of noticing is especially important within our families.

CONFRONTING OUR CURRENT FAMILY PERSPECTIVES

In every family we develop images of each other that we then confirm for ourselves again and again: My older sister is always bossy . . . My dad is always giving me a hard time . . . My husband never notices any-thing . . .

This is what we call the "You Always / You Never" trap. Our experi-ence with our family members starts so early in life that our expectations about relationships become deeply imprinted, and anything that happens, no matter how subtle, often gets pressed into that old imprint. We have to remember that as we grow and change throughout our lives, so do our family members; by not giving them the benefit of the doubt, we may not see how they have changed.

My dad actually called me today—he always expects me to be the one to reach out, that's a big step for him.

My daughter helped her brother with his homework tonight. I wouldn't have expected that, I'll make sure to thank her.

My mother-in-law hasn't always been there for me, but she came through when my child was sick recently. It seems like she's trying, and that's important.

In Chapter Five we mentioned a meditation instruction that's useful in enhancing our everyday ability to notice and pay attention to the world, and this meditation is equally useful when we interact with our families. It is to ask ourselves the question: *What's here that I've never noticed before?*

It can be asked about a relationship just as easily as it can be asked about an environment. *What is there about my relationship with this per-son that I've never noticed before? What have I been missing?*

When you go to Thanksgiving dinner and have to sit next to your brother-in-law who constantly insists that everyone should learn to write computer programming code, or you find yourself cornered by an aunt who wants to talk only about her pet Bichons, try making that question your mantra, at least for the first few minutes (a person can only do so much). *What is there about this person that I've never noticed before?* You might be surprised by what you discover.

One thing we can be sure of—nobody we encounter in life can ever be fully known. There is always more to discover. Making those discoveries, and taking them to heart, can sometimes correct biases that have been stifling our relationships with the people we've known the longest—our families.

FAMILY RELATIONSHIPS: WHY THEY'RE WORTH THE TROUBLE

Sometimes it seems like our families are more permanent than they are; we think our families will always be with us and will always be the way they are now. But as each family member passes into new life stages, the roles we play shift, and *it's often when those shifts happen without our noticing that family problems begin to develop.* Adolescents don't need the same attentiveness they required at age two. Parents or grandparents need more help in their 80s than in their 60s. New mothers may need a family member's help, but not their advice. Sometimes we may need to ask ourselves: *What's an appropriate role for me to play with this person at this stage of our family life?*

Each of us has different knowledge, abilities, and sets of experiences, and these different forms of family "wealth" can be drawn upon when changes occur. A brother who overcame bullying as a child may be able to help your young son who's experiencing the same thing. But to take advantage of these forms of wealth, we have to stay in touch with each other. And we may need to *ask* for that help, to ask for a change in roles.

In addition to new challenges caused by shifting roles, families can drift apart as time passes, for reasons both big and small. Even a small disagreement can lead to neglect that then leads to the end of an important family relationship. When one family member moves away, the inconvenience of visits can mean that the entire family rarely gets together. Recall the how-much-time-is-left relationship equation from Chapter Four—for a family member who rarely comes around, a family's time with that person may add up to only a few days over the course of the rest of their lives. Keeping connections going takes effort. If the reason for disconnection is not geographic, but emotional, then maintaining connection might mean developing a willingness to face feelings of guilt, sadness, or resentment.

The complex emotional lattice of every family is unique in important ways, and our families affect us in ways that other relationships do not. Families share history, experience, and blood as no other relationships can. We can't replace a person we've known for our entire lives. More importantly, we can't replace a person *who's known us* for our entire lives. Nurturing and enriching these relationships despite challenges, persevering, and appreciating the positive things we get from them is worth the trouble. Bob thinks of a moment when, as a young man, he was going through a time in which he was incredibly angry at his parents, and an uncle took him aside. *I know you're mad*, his uncle said. *But just remember: nobody is ever going to care about you this much ever again.*

THE PATH AHEAD

Earlier in this chapter, we offered some pointers for leaving yourself open to those unexpected corrective experiences that can happen with family members when you least expect them. But we can also be proactive in strengthening family connections. Of course, what works for one family may not work for another. But there are some general principles that can help cultivate strong bonds for both immediate and extended families. Here are a few things to think about:

First, start with yourself. What kinds of automatic reactions do you have to your family members? Are you passing judgment based on past experiences, and foreclosing the opportunity for something different to happen?

One simple thing we can all do is to *notice when we find ourselves wanting someone to be different than they are.* We can ask ourselves, *What if I just let this person be themselves without passing judgment? How would this moment be different?* Recognizing another person for *who they are* and meeting them *where they are* can go a long way toward deepening a connection.

Second, routines are important. We mentioned in Chapter Seven that one way to enliven intimate relationships is to step out of routines. While breaking up routines can also be great for families who find themselves stuck in the doldrums, the fact is that *family relationships are often defined by their regular contact.* This is true for families that live under the same roof together, and it's especially true for families that are living apart. Regular get-togethers, dinners, phone calls, and text messages all serve, in combination, to glue a family together. As life changes and becomes more complicated, *finding new rituals can help keep family connections alive* when they would otherwise wither. Regular contact used to happen more often through religious events like baptisms, Ramadan, and bar/bat mitzvahs. These still occur of course, but as the world becomes more secular, some families struggle to find replacements.

Social media tools can help here. Some families that would otherwise drift apart might do well to create more regular contact online. Videoconferencing software is especially powerful, because it allows for more communication through facial expression and body language. Particularly during the Covid-19 pandemic lockdowns, videoconferencing was a lifesaver for many families.

We'd do well to remember, however, that there is always the danger that relying on social media and video calls can create the illusion that we're maintaining *significant* contact, when in fact it's more superficial. There are mysterious and subtle currents of feeling that pass between two people who are physically present with each other. The late night, intimate conversations that Rachel DeMarco described having with her father, Leo, in Chapter Five might not have happened had she not been there in the room with him, the lights dimmed, the family cat on her lap.

There also might be some overlooked opportunities to connect with our immediate families during daily routines. One of the most powerful of these routines happens to be one of the simplest, and the oldest: family dinners.

Any excuse to gather the family together and talk is a good excuse, and there is evidence that it might be especially beneficial for kids. Researchers have found that regular family dinners are associated with children's higher grade-point averages and higher self-esteem, along with lower rates of substance abuse, teen pregnancy, and depression. There is also evidence that eating at home more often leads to healthier dietary habits. Some cultures make meals a centerpiece of family life, but in the Western world, people are eating more meals alone than ever before, with adults in the U.S. eating about half of their meals alone. That is a lot of missed opportunity for connection. Family dinners are a regular opportunity to check in with everyone and keep family members up to date on one another's lives. Even if some of us are annoyed at the routine, it can have the important effect of making everyone feel like they aren't on their own. Adults can model for young children the rules of turn-taking in conversation, sharing, and listening to others' experiences with curiosity, and adults can learn from their kids about cultural trends. And don't underestimate the importance of being together, even if there's not always great conversation. Sometimes important information is conveyed not by what our family members say, but by how it *feels* to be in a room with them. Texts and shouts between rooms have a hard time competing with what we communicate in even fifteen minutes of sitting together at a table. If your family's schedule doesn't allow for dinners, then breakfasts might serve the same function. Every human being needs to eat. As often as we can, we should do it together.

Finally, *remember that every member of the family has their own store of buried treasure*, unique things that only they can provide to the family but that may be hidden in plain sight. Consider, for example, the grandparents who have accumulated entire lifetimes of experience. Their sense of generational identity, of how family members overcame major challenges in the past, and their fund of knowledge about family history can give us perspectives on the present day that are not available through other means. Family stories are important for bonding and maintaining connections. What are the questions you want to ask your aging family members now, before it's too late? What do you want to share with your kids? Asking older relatives for stories about the family can be a way to keep people connected. Short videos, films, and photos can matter a lot, especially after people have passed away. New ways to preserve family history and connection are arising all the time—it benefits us to take advantage of them.

It's not only older generations whose memories are valuable. If you have siblings, their memories of growing up can enrich your own. If your kids are grown, asking them what they remember about their childhood can give you a new perspective on them and on your own experiences as a parent. Shared memories deepen connections.

The Harvard Study, in a way, is a massive experiment in this kind of family inquiry. When we open up an individual file and get that nostalgic feeling of looking through a family photo album, we do it in the spirit of investigation. But you don't need grant funding and the support of an academic institution to mine the treasures that are there in your own family. It takes only curiosity and time. You might find some surprises, good and bad, that enrich your understanding of your family.

Neal McCarthy's kids took advantage of his memory in this way, and had several conversations with their father about his early life. He didn't tell them everything—not as much, it seems, as he told the Harvard Study—but he told them enough for them to know that he'd had both some great times and some incredibly hard times.

In the end, the most important thing was something they saw firsthand: when he formed a family of his own, he didn't run from challenges, he didn't perpetuate the things that made his childhood hard, and he gave his family the gift of his steady presence. Even if he made mistakes, he didn't turn away from them. He was there. When asked what advice she would give to the future generation, his daughter Linda gave an answer inspired by her father, telling the Study, "I'd just say never forget what this life is truly about. It's not about how much money you make. That's what I learned from my dad. It's about the person he was to me, to my child, my sisters and my brother, his seven grandchildren. If I can be half that I'll be all right."

THE GOOD LIFE AT WORK

Investing in Connections

> Judge each day not by the harvest you reap but by the seeds you plant.
>
> William Arthur Ward

Harvard Study Questionnaire, 1979:

Q: If you could stop working without loss of income, would you? What would you do instead?

Over the next twenty-four hours, billions of people across the world will wake up and go to work. Some will head off to jobs that they've strived toward for their entire lives, but most will have little or no choice about the type of work they do, or about the amount of money they make doing it. The purpose of working, for most people, is primarily to provide for themselves and their families. Henry Keane, one of the Harvard Study's inner-city Boston participants, worked in an automobile factory in Michigan for most of his life—not because he loved to build cars, but because it provided a decent living. He grew up poor, and he started working early in life. He did not receive the same advantages that Harvard-educated men like John Marsden (Chapter Two) or Sterling Ainsley (Chapter Four) received, and he didn't make nearly as much money. Yet Henry was by any measure happier in his life than either John or Sterling. Like Henry, most of the other inner-city Study participants had fewer career choices, worked harder jobs, made less money, and retired at a later age than the Harvard men. These elements of their work certainly had an effect on their health and ability to flourish. And yet, Harvard-educated participants' better pay and greater status was no guarantee of a flourishing life. There are many participants in the Harvard Study who held "dream jobs"—from medical researchers to successful authors to wealthy Wall Street brokers—who were nonetheless unhappy at work. And there are inner-city participants who held "unimportant" or difficult jobs and yet derived much satisfaction and meaning from them. Why? What is the missing piece?

In this chapter we focus on one important aspect of work that many of us, regardless of what we do for a living, often overlook: the impact that our relationships at work have on our life. Not only because these relationships are important to our well-being, as we've discussed, but also because they're aspects of our work lives that we have some control over, and that have the potential to improve our daily experience immediately. We may not always get to choose what we do for a living, but making work *work* for us may be more possible than we think.

TWO DAYS IN THE LIFE

Let's imagine a couple of days in the life of a worker, we'll call her Loren, who's experiencing a number of common challenges the two of us see often, both in the lives of research participants and in our clinical work.

For the last six months, Loren has had a job at a medical billing office that handles several doctors' practices. Her coworkers, seated in cubicles around her, are good people, but she doesn't know them very well. Each day the thing she wants most is to finish her accounts and head home, where an entirely different set of challenges awaits. Unfortunately, ending the day on time has been difficult recently because her company has just taken on a new set of accounts, and for months her supervisor has been shuffling his own work onto Loren's desk, giving her unrealistic deadlines and blaming her for working too slowly. Today her supervisor goes home an hour early. She stays two hours late.

When she gets home, her husband and her two daughters, ages nine and 13, are eating dinner. Pizza, for the third time this week. She actually enjoys making dinner for everybody, she enjoys the bustle and catching up with the kids while she cooks, but it hasn't been possible this week, and her husband's strategy is to do the bare minimum. She always asks him to make a salad at least. He hasn't. She doesn't mention it.

Exhausted, her mind spinning, and still in her work clothes, she sits down with them to get in a few minutes of family time.

Her daughters talk about school for a while; she barely hears them. Her husband is scrolling on his phone. She's talked to him before about her looking for a new job—he's for it—but nothing has changed since then, and she doesn't have the energy to rehash that conversation tonight. She's thinking about everything left undone at work and how she'll probably have to stay late tomorrow. Her oldest daughter asks if Loren can drive her to Minneapolis this weekend to shop for . . . Loren cuts her off—"Let's talk about that on Friday," she says, "when my brain is working again." After the pizza is gone, everybody leaves the table. She didn't even get a slice. She eats some leftover crust and makes a bowl of soup for herself. It's been a day much like any other day. Tomorrow the process will start over.

It makes sense that we think of our work lives and our real lives as separate things. Like Loren, many of us feel that the two things exist in entirely different spheres of experience. We work in order to live. Even those of us who are fortunate to be able to do work that we're passionate about often think of the two spheres as separate, and we struggle to find the right balance between work and life.

But are we missing something here? Is the separation we perceive between work and life helping or hindering us in our quest for the good life? What if the value of work—even work we dislike—lies not just in getting paid, but also in the moment-to-moment sensations of being alive in the workplace, and the feeling of vitality we get from being connected to others? What if even the most ordinary workday presents real opportunities for improving our lives and our sense of being connected to the broader world?

The next day Loren's coworker Javier seems stressed out. More than her, even. He sits at his desk with his headphones on, but she can hear him sighing to himself, and he keeps checking his phone. Loren and Javier aren't close, but she asks if everything is okay.

Yesterday he was in a car accident. It was his fault. Everyone is fine, but his car is in bad shape, and his insurance only covers liability. There's no way he can afford a new car, or even to fix this one, and the office is too far away to get there without a car. He'd gotten a ride from his roommate today, which is not a permanent solution.

"Does the car still drive?"

"Barely—I can't take it on the highway."

"My husband is a body mechanic and does rally racing stuff. If you can get it to my house, he'll knock it together for cheap, at least make it drivable."

"I don't think I can afford it."

"It'll be cheap or free if you don't care how it looks. You might have to buy a couple parts and a case of beer. Trust me, this man could build a car out of a pile of garbage. Bring it over. He owes me."

They get to talking, really for the first time. They've worked beside each other for months but assumed they had nothing in common. She's fifteen years older, he's into video games, and mostly they've kept to themselves. Loren mentions how slow her work is going. Javier is a regular in the online forums that discuss the somewhat outdated software they are using. He asks what she's having trouble with and immediately sees that a key part of her work can be automated using the software.

"Give me a minute," he says, and sits down at her station. Ten minutes later, the software is handling work that would have taken her hours. Loren almost breaks into tears of relief.

It turns out they both have a complaint about the physical filing system, which is an entire wall of the office, and sometimes makes their work more difficult. Javier says he recently worked in a similar office where they did the filing differently.

Together they approach the boss and convince him that a change in the filing could make a big difference in productivity. He agrees and tasks the two of them with developing a plan for how to make it happen without disrupting everything. It will have to be done in stages, after regular hours, and it will be a lot of work. But if he okays the plan, they'd get some overtime.

The next day, when Loren comes into the office, a paper sack is on her desk. It's a loaf of sourdough bread. Javier has a family starter that's generations old. She's shocked that this young kid bakes his own bread.

"There's more where that came from," he says.

That night Loren ends up working a bit late again, but not as late as she has been, so she calls her husband and tells him to wait on dinner—she'll be making BLTs with the sourdough.

Several important things happened here. First, Loren turned a coworker into an unlikely friend. The teamwork that flowed from that budding connection, the shared experience, immediately diminished her level of stress. Now they were in the trenches *together*. She didn't just feel relief from receiving help, she felt relief from *offering* help.

Second, a meaningful project developed. This livened up the daily routine, and the results of that project would make her own work life better and easier. She was now an active participant in her office environment, working toward a small goal of her own design. The events that unfolded also connected an achievement to a *relationship*. This is a crucial point. Achievement is most meaningful when it is *relational*. When what we do matters to other people, it matters more to us. We might do something as a team that gives us a sense of belonging, like Loren and Javier, or we might do something that directly benefits others; both are a kind of social benefit. There's also the satisfaction we get from sharing our personal success with friends and family: another benefit.

Finally, Loren's growing friendship with Javier created the possibility that her *work* could become a more meaningful piece of her *life*. The offer to enlist her husband's help and the gift of bread may seem like one-time gestures, but in fact, such gestures open an important door between two worlds—a door that lets positive elements of life flow into work, and vice versa.

We rarely get to choose our coworkers. But while that might seem like a downside of work, it also creates new opportunities for people who may never have the opportunity to meet outside of work to forge unique relationships and a type of understanding that wouldn't be possible otherwise. Despite differences, coworkers like Javier and Loren can experience a meeting of the minds.

WORK VS. LIFE? OR JUST . . . LIFE?

All over the world, adults spend a major proportion of their lives working. There are differences among countries because of economic, cultural, and other factors, but regardless of the country, work still accounts for a significant piece of most people's waking hours.

On average, workers in the United Kingdom do not work the most hours each year (among sixty-six countries polled in 2017, that status belongs to Cambodia) but they don't work the fewest hours, either (that status belongs to Germany), so individuals from the U.K. are good examples of the average worker. By the time the average individual in the U.K. reaches 80 years of age, he or she will have spent about 8,800 hours socializing with friends, about 9,500 hours in activities with an intimate partner, and more than *112,000 hours* (13 years!) at work. People in the United States apportion their time in similar ways. At any one time, 63 percent of all Americans age 16 and over are part of the paid labor force, and there are many more who do important unpaid work like raising children and caregiving for loved ones. That adds up to hundreds of millions of hours of work every day.

When they reached their 70s and 80s, some Harvard Study participants expressed regret about how much time they had spent at work. There's the old cliché that on their deathbeds, no one ever wishes they'd spent more time at the office. It's a cliché for a reason: it's often true:

I wish I had spent more time with family. I worked a lot, just like my father, who was a workaholic. Now I'm worried my son is one, as well.

James, age 81

I wish I'd spent a lot more time with my kids, and less time at work.

Lydia, age 78

I probably worked harder than I should have. I did good work, but it took a lot from me. I didn't take vacations. I gave too much of myself.

Gary, age 80

This is something many of us struggle with. We need to work and to provide for our families, but work tends to pull us away from our families. You might expect a book like this to advocate leaning away from work to focus more on family and relationships, and in many cases, working less might be exactly what someone needs. But the complicated interplay among work, leisure, relationships, home life, and well-being suggests more nuanced solutions. Our time at work affects our time at home, our time at home affects our time at work, and it is our relationships in both places that form the foundation of that interplay. When there is an imbalance, the source can sometimes be found in the way we have been attending to our relationships on one side or the other.

Michael Dawkins, a construction engineer and Study participant, had that common experience of regretting the amount of time he spent working, despite the fact that he took great pride in his work and considered it the central purpose of his life. "I love to create and learn new things and to see changes in myself," he said. "I find there's meaning in finishing projects, and being recognized for what I do. It gives me a good feeling." And yet, he lamented the way he spent his time at home, and the effects his commitment to work had on his marriage. "You don't always notice what you've missed," he said. "Even when you're home, you're preoccupied. Then one day you turn around and realize it's too late."

But other participants, also dedicated to their work, were able to thrive in the midst of this complexity. Take Henry Keane. Though he never told the Study much about the cars he made, he spoke often about how much he enjoyed the companionship he found at work; he thought of his workmates as a second family. His wife, Rosa, who worked in the city payroll office for thirty years, felt the same way about the people she worked with, and the two of them often hosted huge barbecues for everyone they knew from both jobs. It's hard to imagine that at least one new happy couple didn't come from those barbecues.

Or take Leo DeMarco, our high school teacher, who rejected several promotions to administrative positions in order to continue his work as a teacher because his connections with students and other teachers gave him so much joy. His family often wished he'd spent more time at home, but the time they did spend together was valuable, and the strength of their connection undeniable.

Rebecca Taylor, one of the Student Council Study participants, had a different and equally common experience of this complex interplay of work, home, and relationships. At age 46, circumstances had backed Rebecca into a corner, and she found herself struggling. Recently divorced after her husband abruptly abandoned the family, she was raising two children by herself and working full-time as a nurse at a hospital in Illinois. Her son, 10, and daughter, 15, were both devastated by their father's abandonment, and Rebecca was doing her best to provide some stability in his absence. But between her efforts at home and her responsibilities at work, Rebecca was constantly overwhelmed. It seemed she never had enough time.

"Anything I do, I try to do absolutely as well as I can," she told an interviewer, two years after her husband left. "But right now it's just about keeping my head above water. I've been taking additional classes three times a week to get some additional certifications, so when I come home I only have enough time to make dinner, do my reading, and maybe do some housework before bed. I'm too short with the kids. I know they feel how stressed I am and that doesn't help them. But the job defines my life right now. It has to, we need it financially. It's not a dire circumstance, I don't want to be too dramatic. But it's nonstop and the money is just barely enough. Sometimes I just want to give up."

But Rebecca's kids were also there for her, and that gave her a modicum of strength in what felt like an impossible situation. "Sometimes I'll come home and they'll have already done the laundry, and taken out the trash and gotten dinner started. They're both very active in that way. They know we're all in this together. It's such a relief that they feel that way, and it does make us closer. My son is only 10, so with everything going on he's still very attached to me. He follows me around when I get home and we catch up on the day. He talks my ear off. I do my best to listen to him. Sometimes it's hard if I had a rough day."

The spillover effect that work has on our home lives is an especially common worry. We all have bad days at work. A disagreement with a coworker, a lack of recognition of our contributions, feeling discounted at work because of our gender or some other element of our identity, encountering demands that we can't possibly meet—all kinds of things can lead to roiling emotions that we carry with us when we walk out of our workplace to head home. Or, if our primary duties are at home with children, negative emotions may linger after the kids are put to bed and our seemingly endless chores are ended for the day.

What effect do these daily emotional currents that emerge from work have on the other parts of our life? Our partners and families may have only the barest ideas of what we're feeling when we leave work, but they are often the ones who bear the brunt of the emotion.

COMING HOME UPSET

In the 1990s, just as his relationship with his wife-to-be was getting serious, Marc began to worry about his own work-life balance. He was working more than he ever had, and worried not only that he was losing time with the people he cared about, but also that the time they did spend together was affected by his emotions spilling over from work.

Inspired by these personal concerns—as often happens in psychological research—Marc began to use his time at work to investigate . . . time at work, and its connection to the rest of life. He conducted a study to try to quantify the effects of a difficult workday on intimate relationships.

Committed couples with young children filled out questionnaires at the end of the workday and at bedtime over several days. The study was designed to shed some light on the question: When we come home upset, how does it affect our interactions with our intimate partners?

The findings wouldn't surprise many couples: rough workdays were linked with changes in nightly interactions. For women, a difficult workday was linked primarily with angrier behavior, and for men, primarily with withdrawing emotionally from a partner.

A number of the participants in the study, particularly the men, talked about how they usually leave the stress of work at the workplace. But the study showed that even if we think we leave work at work, our emotions carry over in ways that we may not always recognize. A curt reply to an innocent question, zoning out in front of the TV or computer, a conversation about someone else's problems that is shorter than it should be—we might be surprised how much our emotions from work can color our life at home. When our partners come home upset, however, we tend to place the blame on the partners themselves with the familiar refrain, *Don't take it out on me!*

When feelings from work spill over into a close relationship, there is nothing to do but face those emotions. Some of the techniques we've discussed in Chapter Six (regarding adaptation to emotion) and Chapter Seven (regarding intimacy) may be useful here. The cycle initiated by coming-home-upset often goes something like this: One person comes home upset and is less engaged or patient with family members; that person's partner or children respond in a negative way to the altered behavior; this is followed by a negative response from whoever is upset; the evening goes downhill.

Arresting this cycle is difficult, but it can be done, primarily by directly addressing the emotions involved. We feel what we feel, but we don't need to let emotions have their way with us. If we are the ones coming home upset, we first have to *recognize* and *accept* that we are upset and acknowledge that those feelings come from something that happened during the workday. Once we acknowledge these facts, taking a few moments purposely to sit with the emotions—in the parking lot outside work, during our commute, in the shower at home—and allow ourselves to feel them without judgment, can, counterintuitively, alleviate some of the hard edges. We don't need to rehash all the reasons for the emotions, all of the wrongs that have been perpetrated, and fall into a negative thought spiral. And the opposite tactic—trying to ignore the emotions or hide them from our partner—often increases their intensity and our body's arousal. Instead, our most helpful first step is simply to recognize the feelings and acknowledge them to ourselves.

Consider applying some of the lessons we talked about in Chapter Five (regarding paying attention) as well. When we come home upset, often the only thing on our minds is work. But at that point, there is likely not much we can do about whatever made us upset in the first place. To pull yourself out of an upsetting thought-spiral, try noticing your environment, its sounds, its textures. Ask your spouse, "How was *your* day?" and do your best to listen. Really listen. All of this is easier said than done, of course. It takes practice.

If it's your partner who's coming home upset, and you find yourself on the wrong end of irritability or inattentiveness, some similar strategies may help. If you can keep yourself from immediately returning the negativity, take a step back and be curious about what may be going on for your partner. Take a breath and again ask that simple question, "How was your day?" Or change the usual question to indicate that it's not just automatic: "It seems like you had a hard day. Tell me about what happened."

It's inevitable that we will have hard days at work (or many of them in a row). But can we do something about the reasons we're having those hard days? Sometimes these difficult emotions stem from the nature of the work itself, but just as often they stem from the nature of our relationships at work, whether it's a challenging coworker, a demanding boss, or customers who never seem to be satisfied. Often, we think of these work relationships as set in stone. But they don't have to be. Many of the techniques we've discussed thus far for family and intimate relationships can be applied to work relationships as well. The W.I.S.E.R. model for difficult interactions from Chapter Six can be very useful with workmates, too.

In the case of Victor Mourad, one of our inner-city Boston Study participants, the stress he experienced came not from difficult interactions at work, not from a demanding boss, but from a problem that is endemic in the modern workplace: a lack of meaningful interaction. In other words, workdays full of loneliness.

A DIFFERENT KIND OF POVERTY

Victor grew up in the North End of Boston, the son of Syrian immigrants. His was one of several Arabic-speaking families in the Study. The North End was a heavily Italian neighborhood, a fact that often made Victor feel out of place as a child. In every interview over the course of his life, he struck Harvard Study interviewers as both highly intelligent and chronically self-conscious. In fact, he believed that he was less intelligent than almost everyone he met. When he was a kid, if a fellow student played hooky or ran away from home, he believed it was because that student was too smart for school, or more courageous than he was.

"Victor is a frank, open, and lovable boy who attends to everything around him," one of his junior high school teachers told the Study. "But he's a bundle of nerves." After Victor worked a number of odd jobs through his 20s, his cousin started a small trucking company servicing

New England and offered Victor a job. Victor declined, but after he married, and his cousin's company began to do well and expand to multiple locations, Victor reconsidered.

"I figured, well, I like to spend time alone. Driving a truck doesn't sound so bad," he said.

After several years, Victor became a partner in the company, sharing in profits while continuing to drive. He was proud that he made a decent living and maintained a high quality of life for his wife and kids, but that pride did not mitigate his feelings of isolation. He would sometimes be away from home for days at a time and didn't have any real friends that he interacted with on a regular basis. The one person at work he knew well— his cousin—had a short temper, and they often disagreed about how the company should be run. Twenty years after he began the job, he told the Study that the money he earned had prevented him from trying something else, but the job had become a real burden on his life. "If I had any guts I'd quit," he told a Study interviewer. "But a guy like me can't quit because of the economic bag I'm in. I feel like I'm on a treadmill to oblivion."

Like Victor, many of us don't always have a choice about the work we do. Life circumstances and financial need can diminish our options, and it's common to find ourselves stuck in jobs that are not entirely satisfying. It's no coincidence that many of the least satisfying jobs are also some of the loneliest. In the recent past, truck driving, night security, and certain kinds of overnight shift work have been some of the more isolating jobs. Now isolating jobs are also common in emergent, tech-driven industries. People who work for package- and food-delivery services, and other businesses in the gig economy for example, often have no coworkers at all. Online retailing is now a vast industry with millions of workers, but even packing and sorting in a fulfillment warehouse, where there are plenty of coworkers, can be lonely. The work is so fast and furious and the warehouses so vast that many workers on the same shift may not even know each other's names, and there's little opportunity for meaningful interaction.

And of course, there is the foundational and age-old work of raising children; a job that can be as difficult and isolating as any other. Hours of no adult conversation, every day, can be mind-numbing.

If we feel disconnected from others at work, that means we feel lonely for the majority of our waking hours. This is a health concern. As we've mentioned elsewhere, loneliness increases our risk of death as much as smoking or obesity. If we find ourselves feeling lonely at work, it may be up to us to create opportunities for social connection to the extent that we can. For parents raising their kids at home, play dates or visits to a local park (which are often as much for the parents as for the kids) can be restorative. For warehouse workers, there may be opportunities to connect with people directly before a shift, or directly after. For a gig worker, small interactions with others can be opportunities for positive feelings and moments of relief from loneliness (in Chapter Ten, we'll talk more about the importance of these "lesser" interactions). If we want to maximize our well-being at work, we may have to be thoughtful and intentional about it.

However, loneliness at work does not afflict only those who work in solitary jobs. Even busy people with extremely social jobs can feel incredibly lonely if they don't have meaningful connections with their coworkers and colleagues.

The polling firm Gallup has conducted workplace engagement polls for thirty years, and one of their questions that has stimulated the most controversy is: *Do you have a best friend at work?*

Some managers and employees find the question irrelevant or absurd, and in some workplaces, good friendships at work are looked at warily. If employees are chitchatting and seem to be having a good time together, some think that means they're not working and their productivity is probably suffering.

In fact, the opposite is true. *Research has shown that people who have a best friend at work are more engaged than those who don't.* The effect is especially pronounced for women, who are twice as likely to be engaged in their jobs if they "strongly agree" that they have a best friend at work.

When we are searching for jobs, and looking at pay and health benefits, the question of work relationships doesn't often appear. But these connections are themselves a kind of work "benefit." Positive relation-ships at work lead to lower stress levels, healthier workers, and fewer days when we come home upset. They also, simply, make us happier.

UNLEVEL PLAYING FIELDS: INEQUITIES AT WORK AND HOME

Seeking positive relationships at work comes with its own pitfalls, how-ever, and workplaces have historically come with added burdens and chal-lenges for groups that have been marginalized by society. In the early part of the twentieth century in Boston, the marginalized included the immi-grants from poor areas in Europe and the greater Middle East who made up a large proportion of the inner-city sample. It also included the women who were part of the Student Council Study, and today it includes women and people of color who face continuing barriers at work. It's difficult to engage in authentic relationships when there are pervasive power imbal-ances and prejudices.

"I'm worried right now," Rebecca Taylor, the Student Council Study participant mentioned earlier, told an interviewer in 1973, "because the hospital is about to let several nurses go, and I could be one of them. I overheard a conversation the other day among several male doctors, all of them agreeing that it was no big deal if they let any nurses go because they had double incomes with their breadwinner husbands at home. I inter-rupted them! I had to! I said, *Come on guys! You have no idea what you're talking about! You act as if we have no responsibilities at all, as if everyone's situation is the same.* That really infuriated me. This is the kind of think-ing I have to deal with, and for all I know the administrators agree. I could easily lose my job. I don't know what I'll do then."

As a female psychologist in a field dominated by men, Mary Ains-worth (the creator of the Strange Situation procedure used to illuminate a child's attachment style that we discussed in Chapter Seven) had her own encounters with sexism in the workplace. In the early 1960s, she and her other female colleagues at Johns Hopkins University were forced to eat in a separate lunchroom from the men, and she did not receive compensation equal to that of her male counterparts. Earlier in her life she was told that she was not hired for a research position at Queen's University in Canada because she was a woman. The field of psychology—and even this book—would look very different if she hadn't managed to persevere.

A lot of progress has been made on this front in many workplace cultures around the world, but inequities remain. In America, women's roles in the workforce have changed significantly since the 1960s, with women working a larger variety of jobs than ever before, and for more hours. But there has not been a corresponding change in women's roles in the home. In her 1989 book, *The Second Shift*, Arlie Hochschild demonstrated that while there had been a revolution in women's roles in the workplace, women's responsibilities at home remained largely the same, especially among couples that have children.

More than thirty years later, these imbalances in family-rearing responsibilities continue to endure and show up frequently in couples therapy. Men often believe they are contributing equally at home (and certainly doing more than their fathers ever did), when in many cases their contributions of time to home care activities are less than they imagine. A woman might cook dinner, a man might load the dishwasher; one takes an hour, the other takes a few minutes. A woman might help a child with homework, a man will read the child a story before bed. One takes half an hour, the other fifteen minutes. Every relationship is different, but statistically, the time burdens in the home still often weigh more heavily on the woman.

The difficulty for women doesn't end when they leave the house. The Me Too movement has drawn needed attention to sexual abuse and harassment connected to hierarchies and power imbalances in the workplace. But even at a more innocuous level, when sex is not involved, cultivating authentic relationships with others who are at different levels of authority is risky, and this is true for both women and men. Power discrepancies have a tendency to skew and sometimes corrupt all sorts of relationships.

Ellen Freund, the wife of a First Generation study participant, worked in admissions at a university, and she discovered the danger of power imbalances when a particular discrepancy poisoned some of her friendships at work. Asked in 2006 if she had any regrets, she told the Study:

> I do have regrets, actually. It's been a few decades now but I'll tell you about it. Several years after I started at the university I worked with four or five ladies who were about my age. Technically they worked under me, but we became good friends. We socialized all the time. The new dean of admissions asked me to give him a confidential assessment of all the people on the staff—their strengths and their weaknesses. I did this and I was absolutely honest. The office manager thought that I was traitorous. She copied the memorandum and put it on the desk of every one of those ladies. I never thereafter developed a close relationship with anyone that I worked with at the university. And that trails me to this day. It ended my friendships with them. They were pretty good about it. We never talked about it. They realized that what I said was true. I tried my best to be fair. It probably didn't hurt their standing because I said that. But it certainly destroyed my friendships with them.

Asked if she had intentionally avoided forming relationships with others after this incident, Ellen said, "Absolutely. I wanted to be free to deal with people on as nearly pure a professional basis as I could. I didn't want to be influenced or perceived to be influenced by personal relationships."

Ellen chose to disengage from her relationships at work, to separate her "personal relationships" from what she considered her "work relationships." This is a common and understandable strategy. If we minimize our social connections and minimize the degree to which we open ourselves up to our workmates, it will minimize a certain kind of trouble at work. But it can potentially open up new avenues of trouble—including feelings of disconnection and loneliness. In Ellen's case, this decision defined her life at work for the duration of her career, and she eventually came to regret it. What might she have done instead? Facing toward the difficulty—talking with each of her colleagues to see if hurt feelings could be eased—might have allowed her to hold on to at least some of the relationships that she so valued.

These decisions impact the workplace in more ways than one. Not only can disengagement diminish the quality of our time at work, but it can also hinder the transfer of knowledge and stall workers' growth, particularly the growth of younger workers. One of the most valuable types of relationships at work is also one that comes with a power imbalance: that of mentor and mentee.

MENTORSHIP AND THE ART OF GENERATIVITY

When our high school teacher Leo DeMarco was young, he dreamed of becoming a fiction writer. But in the end, that dream gave way to his enthusiasm for teaching, and he found meaning in helping his students pursue their dreams of writing. "Encouraging others," he said, "was more important than doing it myself."

Leo, like all teachers, was in a unique position in that it was his job specifically to be a mentor to his students. But in any profession there are those who are just getting started, and those who've been there a long time. A mentorship relationship can be beneficial for both the mentor and the mentee. As mentors, we get to be generative. It's a very particular joy to be able to extend our influence and wisdom beyond ourselves and into the next generation. We get to pay forward benefits given to us in our own careers—or benefits that we'd always *wished* had been given to us. We also get to enjoy the energy and optimism of people who are at earlier points in their career paths, and to be exposed to fresh ideas that younger people often bring. As mentees, on the other hand, we are able to grow our skills and advance in a career more quickly than if we had to learn everything by ourselves. Some jobs, in fact, require this kind of relationship. There are many jobs in which it is not even possible to learn without some kind of instruction and a close apprenticeship with a more experienced person. Embracing these relationships and cultivating them can make for a much richer experience for everyone involved.

Bob and Marc have benefited from a number of mentors who have shaped our personal careers, and for that matter, our lives. In fact, at different times, we've provided mentorship to each other.

When we first met, Bob was officially Marc's boss, as Bob was the director of the program where Marc was doing his psychology internship. Marc was more than a decade younger than Bob but more advanced in his research training. Soon after they met, Bob decided to apply for a grant that would allow him to pursue research himself. He had an established career as a clinical psychiatrist and educator; doing research would mean leaving his administrative position, and starting from square one. Some of his colleagues counseled against it, saying it was too late, and the transition would be too difficult. Bob went ahead anyway. But he had a problem; a significant part of the grant application included complicated statistical analyses, which were as foreign to Bob as ancient Greek. So he offered Marc both his friendship and a lifetime supply of chocolate chip cookies in exchange for Marc's guidance.

It was a complex relationship: Bob was Marc's boss and had to accept a certain amount of vulnerability in order to ask for help. Marc also was vulnerable, since Bob was substantially senior and had much more security. But we learned from each other. In one direction flowed statistical knowledge, and in the other, a wealth of experience. In the end, Bob got the grant, and made the transition to research (though Marc hasn't seen a cookie from Bob in many years).

As we grow older, and transition from being mentees to being mentors, from students to teachers, new opportunities for connection arise, and those opportunities can come from surprising places. Mentoring younger generations, and sharing wisdom and experience with others, is part of the natural flow of work life, and can make almost any kind of job more rewarding. The satisfaction that comes from being generative makes the good life at work more possible.

WORK TRANSITIONS

As we progress through the stages of our lives there are transitions that will occur in our work as well, whether it be when we receive promotions, get laid off, move into new jobs, or have kids. With each major transition it never hurts to step back and reassess our new lives from a bird's-eye view: *How are my relationships in the work world and beyond being affected by the current change? Are there choices I can make to maintain connections with people who are important to me? Are there new opportunities for connection here that I'm missing?*

One of the most impactful transitions around work is also one of the last: retirement. This is a complicated transition and one filled with relational challenges. The "ideal" retirement—in which a worker puts in the required years on the same job, retires with a full pension, and then lives a life of leisure—has never been that common (and in the modern age is all but extinct).

The Harvard Study asked participants often about retirement. A good number of the men in the study were adamant that their life was too tied up with work to consider the possibility. "I'll never retire!" they said. Some didn't want to retire, others didn't feel financially able to retire, and some were just struggling to imagine a life without work. Some participants' work status was very difficult to pin down. Many refused to think about it, left retirement questions blank when they filled out Study questionnaires, or indicated that they were retired despite the fact that they were continuing to work almost full-time; for them, it seemed, retirement was just a state of mind.

When we retire, it can be a challenge to find new sources of meaning and purpose, but doing so is crucial. Those who fare the best in retirement find ways to replace the social connections that sustained them for so long at work with new "mates." Even if we didn't enjoy working and were doing it only to support ourselves and our family, removing this major organizer of our days can leave an enormous hole in our social lives.

One participant, when asked what he missed about the work he did in his medical practice, which he operated for nearly fifty years, answered, "Absolutely nothing [about the work itself]. I miss the people and the friendship."

Leo DeMarco had a similar feeling. Just after he retired, a Study interviewer visited him at his home and wrote this in his field notes:

> I asked Leo what was most difficult about retirement and he said that he missed his colleagues and said that he tried to stay in touch with them. "I get spiritual sustenance from talking shop." He said he still enjoyed talking about what the task of teaching young people was all about. "It is wonderful to help someone acquire skills." He then told me, "teaching is an almost total human commitment." He said that teaching young people "started the whole process of exploring." He said that small children know how to play and "the adult in education has to remember how to do that." He said it was hard for adolescents and adults to remember how to play because of the other "commitments" in their lives.

Leo was early in his retirement when he said this, and still trying to understand what it meant for him no longer to be teaching. He was looking back on his career, thinking about how it affected him and what it was he was missing, exactly. His comment about adults remembering how to play was something he himself was grappling with; now that work was no longer the center of his life, play could again become important.

For many of us, at a deeper emotional level, work is where we feel that we matter—to our workmates, to our customers, and even to our families—because we are providing for them. When that sense of mattering is gone, we have to find new ways to matter to others. New ways to be part of something bigger than ourselves.

Henry Keane is a representative case. He was abruptly forced into retirement by changes at his factory. Suddenly he found himself with an abundance of time and energy, so he looked for some volunteer opportunities where he felt he could be helpful. First he began working at a nursing home run by Veterans Affairs, and then he started participating in the American Legion and Veterans of Foreign Wars. He was also able to put more time into his hobbies, refinishing furniture and cross-country skiing. But even with all of that, it didn't feel like enough. Something was missing.

"I need to work!" he told the Study at age 65. "Nothing too substantial but I'm hoping to find some jobs that will keep me busy and add to my income. I'm realizing that I just love to work and to be around people."

It wasn't so much that Henry needed the money—he had a decent pension and was happy with that income—it was that earning money would somehow make his activities feel like they mattered; someone was paying him for them. Each person must find their own way of mattering to others.

Henry's realization about wanting to be around people also teaches us an important lesson—not about retirement, but about work itself: the people we work with matter. It's important to look around our work-places and appreciate those coworkers who add value to our lives. Since work is often so shrouded in financial concerns, in stress and worry, the relationships we develop there sometimes don't get their due. We often don't notice how significant our work relationships really are until they're gone.

THE EVOLVING NATURE OF WORK

On the northeast outskirts of Philadelphia, not far from where Marc lives, is a large plot of a land that used to be a family farm. People who lived near the farm could drive by in the morning and see green pastures, with cattle grazing. When World War II began the farm was sold to the U.S. govern-ment and converted into an enormous industrial complex for producing artillery shells and prototype planes. The view changed to buildings and runways, with trucks and planes taxiing. After the war, various types of manufacturing continued on the site until the late 1990s, when it was sold and transformed into a golf course. Homes were built around the course, and people could look out their windows and see trees and fairways and motoring golf carts instead of an industrial park. Now, thirty years later, after further changes in the economy, the golf course was sold, and as this book is being written a large portion of the land is now being converted into a UPS sorting center. Soon, when the people who live nearby look out their windows, the fairways and golf carts will have been replaced by a vast warehouse and delivery vehicles. This area is not unique; all over the country, in every sector of the economy, we are witnessing these evolutions.

Our inner-city Boston participants' most formative years, from when they were toddlers until they reached their preteen years, occurred during the Great Depression. Growing up at a time when they couldn't take financial security for granted shaped how they would go on to conduct their work lives. For them, work was often less about creating a good life, and more about staving off disaster.

The economic trials that those participants experienced are relevant today, when we face economic, environmental, and technological challenges that are causing uncertainty for the foreseeable future. The uncertainty that Henry Keane or Wes Travers would have felt when standing in a Depression-era breadline is directly related to the uncertainty that a Gen Z child might have felt when watching her family evicted from her childhood home during the 2008 financial crisis, or that young people face as we emerge from the Covid-19 pandemic.

Despite technological advances, there are still plenty of people working grueling jobs, people still struggling to meet their basic needs. The idealized prosperity that many expected to arrive with the computer and the information age has been limited to certain sectors and people, leaving others worse off than before. New technologies are changing how often we interact with others at work. Artificial intelligence is replacing some jobs and people with automated systems, creating more interaction with machines and less with human beings. Advances in communication technologies are making remote work much more common for jobs in business, media, education, and other industries, and an always-on mentality threatens to make workers' home lives into an extension of the work sphere. To say the least, a consideration of how these changes have affected our social fitness has not been a top priority. And yet the state of our relationships is among the most important factors in our health and well-being.

In Chapter Five we encouraged you to remember that the time each of us has left is both a finite resource and an unknown quantity. If we want to take full advantage of the hours of our lives—many of which are spent at work—we must remember that *work is a major source of socializing and connection. Change the nature of work, and you change the nature of life.*

The Covid pandemic could not have made this clearer. Millions of people who were locked down in their homes and laid off, furloughed, or forced to work remotely, quickly found themselves missing the connections they were used to having every day. We became isolated from our workmates, customers, and colleagues. Bob and Marc, for example, began using remote tools to teach, work with colleagues, and even to see people in therapy. That took some getting used to. It was better than nothing, but it was not the same as before.

More technological development is inevitable. Because of the economic advantages (the lower cost of not maintaining an office), and advantages of flexible schedules and reduced commutes for employees, more jobs will undoubtedly include remote or partly remote options. This might make sense financially and for certain logistical reasons, but how will it affect the well-being of workers?

The opportunity to work remotely can have positive effects. It allows some workers greater flexibility and more contact with their families. It's especially favorable for working parents who would like to spend more time at home, or who don't have access to or can't afford child care, and to those who have expensive or onerous commutes to work.

But there is a flip side to that coin, as well. Working from home detaches us from important social contact in the workplace. We may feel an initial liberation, and love the new convenience, but as we discussed in Chapter Five, the losses we experience from new technological advances are often veiled by the gains, and these losses are potentially profound. More research is needed, but the loss of in-person contact as we move as much work as possible into the home may have a significant impact on the mental health and well-being of workers. While parents who work from home might get some benefits from being more available to their families, doing so can also place a greater burden on them, forcing them to work and care for children at the same time. And it's likely that this burden will fall harder on working mothers and those with fewer resources for supplemental child care.

As we confront these changes, we can and should ask ourselves the question: How are these technological changes in the workplace affecting our *social fitness*? If automation means we are interacting more with machines and less with people, is there a way to cultivate new social environments at work? If more of us are going to be working remotely, how can we replace the in-person contact we used to get at work?

Our brains, tuned for novelty and danger, catch fire when stimulated by the wonders of new technology and the stresses of the workplace. Compared to those two things, the subtle currents of our positive relationships, so important to our well-being, are likely to be overshadowed. If our relationships—both at work and at home—are going to thrive in this new work environment, we have to elevate and care for them. We are the only ones who can. If we don't, and if the Harvard Study still exists in eighty years, then when today's youngest generation reaches their 80s and the interviewers ask if there was anything they regret about their lives, they might look back, as some of our First Generation participants did in their comments quoted earlier in this chapter, and realize that something crucial has been lost.

MAKING THE MOST OF YOUR WORK HOURS

We often think we have plenty of time to make changes, plenty of time to figure out how to improve our life at work or to balance our work and home life—*If I can only get through this current difficulty, this current issue,*

I'll have time to think about that; there's always tomorrow—but five or ten years can pass in no time. We conducted personal interviews with Harvard Study participants every ten to twenty years. That seems like a long time, but whenever we requested a new interview, participants often said something like, *Has it been that long already?* It seemed to them that a decade had passed in the blink of an eye.

In Chapter Five we talked about the common illusion that there will always be time for the things we need to do, and how in reality we only have the present moment. If we are always imagining that there will be time *later*, one day we'll look around and realize there is no more later. Most of our *nows* will have passed.

So tomorrow when you get up and go to work, consider a few questions:

- Who are the people I most enjoy and value at work, and what is it about them that is valuable? Am I appreciating them?
- Who is different from me in some way (who thinks differently, comes from a different background, has different expertise), and what can I learn from that person?
- If I'm having a conflict with another worker, what can I do to alleviate it? Would the W.I.S.E.R. model be useful?
- What kinds of connections am I missing at work that I might want more of? Could I imagine a way to make these connections more likely, or richer?
- Do I really know my workmates? Is there someone I'd like to know better? How can I reach out to them? You might even pick that person with whom you seem to have the least in common, and make a point to be curious and ask about something that they've displayed, like pictures of family or pets or a T-shirt they wear at work.

Then, when you head home, consider how you feel and how the experiences of the workday might influence your time at home. It could be that this influence is, on balance, a good one. But if not, are there small, reasonable changes that can be made? Would ten minutes or half an hour to yourself help, or a short walk or swim before you get home from work? Would it help to turn your smartphone off for a specific period of time to keep work from spilling into family time?

Sometimes we'd rather be doing anything other than working. But these hours are a major social opportunity. Many of the happiest men and women in the Harvard Study had positive relationships with their work and their workmates, whether they were selling tires or teaching kindergarten or performing surgery, and they were able to balance (often after much difficulty and negotiation) their work lives with their home lives. They understood it was all of a piece.

"When I look back on my work life," Ellen Freund, the university administrator, told the Study in 2006, "I sometimes wish I had paid more attention to the people who had worked for me or around me and less to the problem at hand. I loved my work. I really did. But I think I was a difficult and impatient and demanding boss. I guess I sort of wish—now that you mention it—that I had known everyone a little better."

Our life doesn't wait at the door when we walk into work. It doesn't stand on the side of the road when we climb into the seat of our truck. It doesn't peer through the classroom window as we meet with our students on the first day of class. Every workday is an important personal experience, and to the extent we can enrich each one with relationships, we benefit. Work, too, is life.

ALL FRIENDS HAVE BENEFITS

My friends are my "estate." Forgive me then the avarice to hoard them.

Emily Dickinson

Ananda, one of the Buddha's disciples, said to the Buddha one day, "I've realized that half of the path to the holy life is made of good friendships."

"No, Ananda," the Buddha said. "Friends are not half of the holy life. They are all of the holy life."

Upaddha Suta

Without friends, no one would choose to live.

Aristotle, *Nicomachean Ethics*

Harvard Study Questionnaire, 1989:

Q: Consider your 10 best friends (excluding family and close relatives). How many of them would you place in each of the following categories?
(1) Intimate; we share most of our joys and sorrows;
(2) Companionship; we have frequent interactions arising out of shared interests;
(3) Casual; we don't seek each other out.

When Louie Daly was in his 50s, a Study interviewer asked him about his oldest friend. "I'm afraid I don't have any friends," he said. "The closest friend I ever had was a guy named Morris Newman, we were roommates in my freshman year of college. It was Mo that introduced me to jazz music, which I'm passionate about now. We were extremely close for a year until he flunked out. We wrote back and forth for about ten years after that. Then he stopped writing. Five years ago I thought I missed Mo, so I paid $500 to a search agency to find him. They did actually find him, and we started corresponding again. Then one day about three months later I went out to the box and there was a letter there but it wasn't from Mo. It was from his attorney telling me that Mo had suddenly passed away."

Asked who he would call now if he had a problem, Louie said, "I'm a very self-sufficient person. I don't need people as much."

Leo DeMarco reported a different experience. When asked by an interviewer if he had a best friend, Leo said without hesitation, "Ethan Cecil." They'd known each other since grade school and were still close. Ethan lived a couple of hours away and would drive over now and then, plop himself down, and just start talking. While Leo was discussing this friendship, the phone rang, and Leo spoke with the caller in a very animated voice. When he hung up, he said, "That was Ethan."

What does it mean, in our adult lives, to have a friend? What does it mean to *be* a friend? How important are friendships in our lives, really?

When we're kids, friendships are often central, in part because they have such an intense quality to them. The strength of connection between two friends in childhood (or even in young adulthood) is rivaled only by the intensity of the hurt if the friendship goes wrong. If we feel loved, our hearts soar with a sense of belonging, and if we feel wronged or if we're bullied, those wounds cut deep.

We change as we grow older, and as a consequence our connections to friends change. Friendships that were central during young adulthood may wither away in the early years of a marriage or when children are born, but then go through a resurgence during a difficult period in a marriage, or after the death of a loved one.

All of this is natural. But along with the natural ebb and flow of life, each of us has a habitual approach to friendships. Often this approach is less than conscious, close to automatic. We give our friendships whatever feels natural to give them, rather than considering what they need. As we get older and life becomes busier, we have to make decisions about the limited time we have, and our friends often come last. Responsibilities to family and work may be prioritized over a phone call to an old friend or a coffee with a new friend or a regular card game or a monthly book club (we recommend *The Good Life*). *Sure, it's fun to go out and have a good time with friends*, we might think as we're deciding where our time should go, *but I just have more important things to do.* Or we might think, *My friendships will always be there—I can pick them up again when the kids are older . . . when work slows down . . . when I have some extra time.*

The truth is, our friends are much more important to our health and well-being as adults than we give them credit for. It's amazing, in fact, how powerful the effects of friendships can be on our adult lives, considering the amount of attention they get. Friends can pick us up when we're down, provide an important connection to our own history, and perhaps most importantly make us laugh; sometimes nothing is as beneficial to our health as a good time.

For centuries, philosophers have observed the profound effects of friendship. The Roman philosopher Seneca wrote that the value of friends reaches far beyond what they can do for us. We don't keep friends just to have someone who can sit by our bedside when we're sick, or to come to our rescue when we're in trouble. "Anyone thinking of his own interests and seeking out friendship with this in view is making a great mistake," Seneca wrote. "What is my object in making a friend? To have someone to be able to die for, someone I may follow into exile."

Seneca was speaking to the fact that the benefits of friendships are sometimes obscure and not easily observed. Perhaps because of this, these relationships are often neglected. Good friendships don't always call out to us or stick themselves under our noses, waiting for attention. Sometimes, they just quietly step into the background of our lives and slowly fade away.

It doesn't have to be like this. If we look more carefully, we might find that we've been failing to notice straightforward, potentially fun opportunities to pay attention to friends and awaken our social universe—opportunities that are hiding in plain sight and that could profoundly improve the quality of our lives. Friendships may not *require* our care, but they can't care for themselves.

GOOD COMPANY ON A DIFFICULT PATH

Thirty years ago, when Bob and Marc first met, our connection was primarily professional. Once a week, we'd get lunch and talk about things like statistical models, research methods, and study design. Even though the conversations were mostly about professional matters (and the occasional focus on office politics and other gossipy topics), each of us had a growing sense that the other was a person we wanted to know better. So, even when we had no pressing business, we kept meeting for lunch every week at the same time. And of course, we found more and more to talk about— our families, our hobbies, childhood memories.

At one point, we proposed getting together with our wives for a dinner. Luckily Bob's wife, Jennifer, and Marc's wife, Joan, found that they enjoyed each other's company. Joan and Jennifer had to sit through occasional conversations about statistical analysis, but they accepted that burden and in a relatively short time the four of us had become good—if not yet close—friends. At one point, after a couple of months without a dinner, Bob and Jennifer invited Marc and Joan over. Joan was pregnant for the first time, the due date was just over a month away, and she and Marc were nervously anticipating the birth. Bob and Jennifer already had two young sons of their own, so Marc and Joan were looking forward to getting some reassurance and advice about what to expect.

But at the end of a workday on the Thursday before the scheduled dinner, Marc got a frantic call from Joan. During a routine check-up, the doctor told her she needed to go to the hospital immediately for an emergency C-section. Marc ran out of work, almost crashing into Bob on the way.

"It's Joan and the baby," Marc said. "She's in an ambulance on her way to the hospital."

When Marc arrived, Joan was being connected to monitors and writhing in agony. The doctors explained that she had a life-threatening form of preeclampsia. Her liver was showing signs of failure, her blood pressure, visible on a monitor behind her, was skyrocketing, and she kept asking Marc and the nurses for reassurance that it was beginning to come down. Marc and Joan both remember the doctors saying that Joan and the baby would likely die if the C-section wasn't performed right way.

As they prepped Joan for surgery, Marc called Bob to give him a quick update. Bob let Marc know that he was available at any time to come to the hospital to keep Marc company. The events unfolded too quickly that evening for Bob to make it to the hospital, but in the midst of the most visceral worry Marc had ever experienced, Bob's offer of help was incredibly powerful and reassuring. Both Marc and Joan's families were too far away to make it in time, and a comforting friend was sorely needed.

The C-section went smoothly, and Marc was there with Joan to witness the birth of their son and to share in the relief as Joan's blood pressure began to return to normal. They both rejoiced as their son let out his first cry—really more of a squeak. Born a month early, he was small as a bird (weighing in at four and a half pounds), but otherwise healthy. Joan and Marc were so tired that they could not even decide on the baby's name. Marc gave Bob the update and told him they were going to try to get some sleep.

The next day, Bob canceled his commitments and came to visit Joan, Marc, and the newly named Jacob in the hospital.

Joan's recovery was a slow one, but after five long days they left for home. Marc and Joan have a video of Joan shuffling out of the hospital and Jacob fidgeting in a car seat for his departure. It's not the best quality video—it's a little bouncy—but then Bob isn't the best videographer.

Those days were such a blur for Marc that it wasn't until much later that he thought back on them and realized that having Bob close by, even though there was nothing Bob could do to help Joan, made a real difference. It also showed Marc that their friendship wasn't just about statistics and research and some good times during a few dinner dates. Bob was there for him and Joan when it really mattered. And he knew that when the time came, he would be there for Bob, too.

This is just one of many stories in the life of our friendship; the friendship that has now, twenty-six years later, brought you this book. When you think of the more difficult times of your life, you may have similar stories that come to mind. When adversity strikes—and it eventually does—it is often our friends who help us through, who buffer us against the wild weather of life.

The power of friendship isn't just the stuff of anecdotes or philosophical observation; science has clearly shown this effect. Friends diminish our perception of hardship—making us perceive adverse events as less stressful than we might otherwise see them—and even when we do experience extreme stress, friends can diminish its impact and duration. We feel the stress, but with the help of friends we're better able to manage it. Less stress and better stress management lead to less wear and tear on our bodies.

Friends, in short, keep us healthier.

In Chapter Two we discussed a 2010 review conducted by Julianne Holt-Lunstad and others that brought together 148 studies and a vast amount of data to analyze the effect that social connections have on health and longevity. Among those 148 studies were a number that focused specifically on friendship. Here are a few that make the point:

- A large longitudinal study in Australia found that people over 70 with the strongest network of friends were 22 percent less likely to

die during the study period (ten years) than those with the weakest
network of friends

- A longitudinal study of 2,835 nurses with breast cancer found that
women who had ten or more friends were four times more likely to
survive than women who had no close friends.

- A longitudinal study of over 17,000 men and women between the
ages of 29 and 74 in Sweden found that stronger social connections
decreased the risk of dying from all causes by almost a fourth over
a period of six years.

The list goes on. When we increase our connection to friends, it has a
measurable effect on our bodies because our bodies need what friendships
provide. The human need for friends and the cooperation that comes with
them is an important evolutionary piece of what has made human beings
a successful species. Having friends, having a group that we belong to, has
always made survival in dangerous environments more likely, and friends
also protect our health in stressful modern environments. No matter how
strong we are, how independent we are, how self-sufficient we are, we are
still biologically tuned for friendship. When the going gets tough, even
the tough benefit from having friends.

A TROVE OF HARD TIMES

In some ways, the Harvard Study is uniquely positioned to investigate the
connection between friendship and adversity, because it is a trove of hard
times. All of our First Generation participants lived through the Great
Depression. Almost all of the Boston inner-city cohort came from humble
(to say the least) and sometimes tragic beginnings, and a number of the
Harvard College cohort grew up in challenging economic or social circumstances. In the college cohort, 89 percent fought in World War II,
as we have mentioned, and about half of those were involved in combat. Many of the inner-city participants, who were a few years younger,
fought in the Korean War. Some of the Study participants faced situations

in which they had to kill or be killed, and some witnessed their friends being killed. Some came home with what has since been recognized as post-traumatic stress disorder (PTSD).

What role did friendships play amid these challenges? Do their experiences have any lessons for us?

They do. Using participants' firsthand accounts of their combat experiences and their connections to fellow servicemen, we found that those men who had more positive friendships with their fellow servicemen, and who served in combat units that were more cohesive and connected, were less likely to experience symptoms of PTSD after the war. Their friendships, in other words, were like a kind of protective armor. Having good and trusted friends buffered these men during some of the most difficult events of their lives.

Some of those relationships endured. One of the questions we asked participants was about their later-life contact with the friends they made during the war. Some still exchanged Christmas cards with their fellow servicemen, still spoke on the phone with them occasionally, and even continued to travel to visit them right up to the very end of their lives. Some even reported keeping in touch with the spouses of their military comrades.

Most, however, lost contact with those comrades, just as they'd lost contact with other friends. As their lives went on, challenges kept coming, but they had to weather them without the support of close friends. Like Neal McCarthy (Chapter Eight), there are participants in the Study who served in war, saw combat, but told us that their most difficult experiences occurred during their civilian lives. Divorces, accidents, the deaths of spouses or of children, and other kinds of intense, stressful experiences weighed on them. But as they aged, their attention to friendships often waned, until they found themselves facing stressful experiences without the support of friends. Unlike when they were in combat, they had no peers to turn to or to share their hardships with. No one to help them through.

WITHERING FRIENDSHIPS

Looking through the files of the Study, it doesn't take long to find men who, in their later years, regretted the way their friendships turned out. These include the cases of extreme isolation and loneliness like Sterling Ainsley (Chapter Four) or Victor Mourad (Chapter Nine), but all through the Study run currents of a more common feeling of disconnection, in which men forge ahead through the stages of their adult lives with fewer and fewer close friendships. When given the opportunity to talk about the state of their friendships—an opportunity they rarely had outside of the Study's investigations—these men almost always claimed their lack of close friendships was due to their self-sufficiency and independence. At the same time, many expressed a longing for more closeness with friends.

"Many men like me regret not having had more close friends," one participant told the Study. "I've never had a really close friend. My wife has more friends than me."

Though this experience with friends is common in the Study, particularly for men, there is no strong evidence to support the belief that men are somehow "wired" for emotional independence and stoicism and averse to intimacy. Instead, it's likely that this approach to friendships (and relationships generally) is primarily the result of cultural forces. For example, friendship patterns among LGBTQ+ individuals often differ from those of their heterosexual counterparts, and there are likely to be generational differences in how men conduct their social lives as they age.

Research indicates that differences in friendship patterns between men and women are actually small. A number of longitudinal studies show that male adolescents from many different backgrounds connect intimately with close friends in ways that defy gender stereotypes. For example, psychologist Niobe Way has studied friendships among Black, Latino, and Asian American adolescent and teenage boys who, like our own inner-city participants, grew up in modest circumstances in a major city.

"Secret sharing or talking intimately with best friends was how the boys in my studies defined a best friend," Way wrote. For example,

Mark says in his freshman year: "[My best friend] could just tell me anything and I could tell him anything. Like I always know everything about him. . . . We always chill, like we don't hide secrets from each other. We tell each other our problems." . . . Eddie, a sophomore, says: "It's like a bond, we keep secrets, like if there is something that's important to me like I could tell him and he won't go and make fun of it. Like if my family is having problems or something." While boys spoke about loving to play basketball or videogames with their friends, the emphasis with their best friends was on talking together and sharing secrets.

As boys age into late adolescence and early adulthood, friendships often become more guarded, and less free. Some of this change is in response to changing life circumstances, and occurs for both men and women—jobs and romantic relationships get in the way. But for men there is often an extra set of powerful cultural forces at work. In many cultures around the world, boys are encouraged to display their independence and masculinity as they age, and they begin to worry that emotional closeness to male friends will make them appear less masculine. Over time, certain intimacies between friends are lost.

Adolescent female friendships are certainly subject to many of their own pressures and constraints, but women in many cultures are expected to continue to maintain and nurture these intimate exchanges beyond the teen years. These expectations may help support further intimacy but they may also result in women carrying a heavier burden for navigating and solving emotional challenges in close relationships.

In 1987 the Study sent one questionnaire to the First Generation participants, and, if they were married, a second questionnaire to their wives. One of the things the Study was particularly interested in that year was the couple's experience with friends.

The men were asked, *How satisfied are you with the number of and your closeness to friends (besides your wife)?* Thirty percent said that they were not satisfied and would like much more. When their wives were asked a similar question, only 6 percent said that they were not satisfied.

Around this same time, sociologist Lillian Rubin was doing important work looking at the question of why men and women seemed to experience their friendships differently.

Women, Rubin found, were more likely than men to keep up contact with their friends. The nature of their relationships was also different— men were more likely to organize friendships around activities, women were more likely to be emotionally close, and to share intimate thoughts and feelings with each other. Women had more *face-to-face* friendships, men had more *side-by-side* friendships.

Rubin's observations have found some support in reviews of multiple studies, but as more and more research has been done on this topic, one thing has become clear: *the gender differences between what men and women seek in friendships are smaller than one might expect given our cultural assumptions.*

For example, studies show that women generally have higher expectations than men about having intimate exchanges in their friendships, but this difference is small. In psychology, small differences between groups mean that the overlap among the two groups is the rule rather than the exception. As a whole, research shows that most people regardless of gender identification want and need similar kinds of closeness and intimacy from their friends.

THE FRIENDSHIPS AT THE HEART OF THE HARVARD STUDY

When Study participants receive a questionnaire in the mail, it doesn't just come with a return envelope. It comes with a friendly letter from the Harvard Study staff. Over the years there has been a great deal of correspondence between the staff and the participants, and a quick perusal of these letters in the participants' files reveals the depth of connections that were made. In the minds of First Generation participants, one particular name at the end of those letters came to be synonymous with the Harvard Study: Lewise Gregory Davies.

Trained as a social worker, Lewise joined the Study in its very first days, when Arlie Bock was just beginning the research. As the Study expanded, Lewise became more and more involved in the outreach to participants. They came to know her by name, would write her personal notes with news of their lives (even though their questionnaires covered most details), and if they were late in returning a questionnaire, she would check in with them and offer an encouraging reminder. Lewise saw them as friends, even as a kind of second family. Many of them responded to questionnaires and interview requests out of loyalty to her personally.

Eventually Lewise retired, but after her husband died, she found herself missing the friends she'd made at the Study, so she came back, and continued her work. It was this personal commitment to the Study, from Lewise and from others, that helped keep almost 90 percent of participants engaged in the Study across eight decades. Our participants knew that they mattered not only to the Study and to the research—most of which they would never see—but to Lewise. In 1983, after she retired for the second time, Lewise wrote a short note to all the participants in the Study, thanking them a final time for one of the defining experiences of her life:

Dear Friends,

Through these many years I have treasured my friendship with you and your families. The memories have been like a shining light in my life. Your loyalty and devotion to the Study have touched me deeply. May the years ahead be rich in happiness and fulfillment for you and those you love,

Devotedly, your old and good friend,

Lewise

This was a relationship that might have seemed unimportant. Many of the participants met Lewise in person only once or twice, and some may have never met her. But she was a part of their lives, and many were happy to have known her. Even though it may have seemed a small, insignificant relationship, in truth it was anything but. Like Rosa Keane in Chapter Nine, Lewise cultivated strong connections at work and grew personally in the process. Were it not for all of these small connections, and the fleeting but positive feelings that came with them, the Harvard Study would probably not be here today.

THE IMPORTANCE OF "UNIMPORTANT" RELATIONSHIPS

Henry Keane, Rosa's husband, when asked for his definition of a true friend, gave an answer that many of us would probably agree with:

"A true friend is someone you can always count on for companionship or for help if you need it."

This is the kind of friendship that social scientists would call a "strong tie." These are the people we know will be there for us when things go wrong, who lift us up when we're down, and who we are prepared to support in their times of trouble. When most of us think of "important friends," these are the relationships that come to mind.

But a relationship doesn't need to be one of our most frequent or intimate contacts to be valuable. In fact, few of us realize that *some of our most beneficial relationships can be with people we don't spend a lot of time with or don't know very well.* Even interactions with complete strangers carry hidden benefits.

Consider the most common and simplest of interactions: buying a cup of coffee. When you go into the coffee shop, how often do you talk to the server? How often do you ask with genuine interest how they're doing, or how their work is going that day? You may or may not be in the habit of doing this, but either way, most of us probably wouldn't think of these interactions as "important." Is that true? Do these interactions matter at all?

In one fascinating study, researchers divided a set of participants (who wanted a coffee) into two groups: one group was instructed to have an interaction with the barista, and the other to be as efficient as possible. Like the "strangers on a train" study that we mentioned in Chapter Two, the researchers found that people who smiled, made eye contact, and had a social interaction with the barista—in this case, a complete stranger— came away feeling better, and with a greater sense of belonging, than those who were instructed to be as efficient as possible. In short, having a friendly moment with a stranger was uplifting.

Small moments can provide an uplift for our mood and they can help balance out some of the stress we feel. An annoying commute can be softened by a short conversation with the security guard at work. A sense of disconnection can be alleviated when we say hello to our mail carrier. These kinds of minute interactions can affect our mood and energy throughout the day. If we get in the habit of seeking out and noticing opportunities for these daily uplifts, over time they can have far-reaching effects. Not only for us, but for our social networks as a whole; repeated casual contact has been shown to foster the formation of closer friendships. And sometimes even the most casual contact can open us up to whole new realms of experience.

THE LONG REACH OF "WEAK" TIES

Casual friendships may be the most overlooked relationships we have. They neither take up the most time nor impact our lives in the most obvious ways. But there is now a great deal of research into the benefits of these connections (which social scientists refer to as "weak ties"—not our favorite term since sometimes there's nothing weak about them). These are the relationships we may not turn to when we're in distress, but that nonetheless provide us with jolts of good feeling or energy during our days, as well as a sense of connection to larger communities.

The sociologist Mark Granovetter has done important research showing the crucial significance of these casual ties. People we know only peripherally, Granovetter has argued, create important bridges to new social networks. These bridges allow for the flow of different and often surprising ideas, the flow of otherwise unavailable information, and the flow of opportunities. Granovetter has shown, for example, that people who cultivate casual ties are more likely to find better work. When you increase the complexity of a social system, a wider variety of things can happen. Casual ties can also lead to a more expansive sense of our own community. The more we talk to people outside of our bubbles, connect with them and humanize our experiences with them, the more empathic we can be when conflicts arise.

Look at your "social universe" chart from Chapter Four. Or, if you didn't make a chart, just think for a moment about your friend universe, and the kinds of interactions you have on a daily basis. Do you have relationships that connect you to other social groups? How about friends that expose you to new or different ideas? Are there opportunities to cultivate some of the "weak" ties in your social universe?

These casual relationships are also the most changeable; they often drift in and out as our lives change. Harvard Study participants' connections to Lewise Gregory and the Harvard Study staff were maintained because of years of systematic effort and devotion; most distant or casual relationships don't get that kind of attention.

In Chapter Three we talked about the ways that our relationships change as our position in the lifespan changes, and this is especially true for friends. Often, gaps in our map of friendships open up because our lives no longer easily accommodate a certain kind of relationship. We've morphed from young adults who had time to hang out with friends most evenings and weekends into parents of small children with hardly a moment to ourselves. Or we've transitioned from busy workdays filled with meetings with coworkers to the long-awaited freedom of retirement where we find ourselves suddenly more alone than we expected. As we move through life, our social lives don't always keep pace.

DIFFERENT FRIENDS FOR DIFFERENT TIMES (FRIENDS THROUGH LIFE STAGES)

Take a walk through your town or neighborhood on a summer day and you might see slices of friendship among people at every stage of life: adolescent boys and girls playing team sports; middle-aged adults meeting for coffee or out for a run together; a group of parents at a playground, all with toddlers and children about the same age; octogenarians meeting for a game of chess in the park.

Our stage of life has a major impact on the role that friendships play and the types of friendships we have. New friendships often arise out of particular life situations, and they can also help us navigate those situations.

Adolescents find connections through discovering new things together and sharing their thoughts and feelings. College students, wrapped up in the intense experience of being on their own for the first time, bond over common challenges, developing trust in each other along the way. New parents thirst for firsthand information about childrearing and look for people who know what they're going through, who they can turn to for both emotional and practical support (Marc and Joan, by the way, continued to rely on Bob and Jennifer for this support, including for some babysitting so they could enjoy their first date night after Joan recovered). And as we have discussed, giving help can be as important to our well-being as receiving it, so parents at a more advanced stage (as Bob and Jennifer were) benefit from *providing* that type of support. Life-stage-specific connections can be strong because these friends have gone through something powerful together. When life changes again, as it always does, these friendships may fade. But sometimes even a short period of intense connection can forge friendships that last for decades and endure through many other life stages.

We don't always go through life stages in lockstep with our friends. We may have friends who were in sync with us in the past but who suddenly seem out of step with our lives right now. If we want to maintain those connections, we may have to work harder to bridge the gap, and to understand what those friends' lives are like.

This happens all the time with people who have not found a partner, but whose friends are already married and having kids. Suddenly these single adults find themselves in a different world. Now conversations revolve around babies and diapers, and the friends without children can feel left behind. It may not be so much about feelings of jealousy as about loss of a connection that seemed as though it might be there, in the same way, forever.

But with every passage from one life stage into another, it's natural that certain friendships will be lost. One common theme among a huge number of Study participants, both women and men, is the loss of friends after retirement. As we discussed in Chapter Nine, for some of us work is the foundation of our social universe. When it's removed, our social fitness can suffer.

This happened to Pete Mills, one of our college participants. Once he retired from his career as a lawyer, he realized with some concern that his entire social life had been built around his work and that he needed to be proactive in rebuilding his social connections. In an effort to find some new friends, he and his wife took up bowling.

"I asked how much entertaining they did," a Study interviewer wrote in her field notes.

Monday night, he said, they had had 20 for "drinks and heavy appetizers" after bowling. Friday night they had had 6 for dinner. He does the floors. She dusts.

I asked what the two of them did together that brought them the most joy. "We do a lot of socializing," he said. The bowling group gets together once a month. They have a play reading group that also gets together regularly. "She doesn't read loud enough. I do," he said mischievously.

I asked about connections with people outside the family. "We do a lot of connecting," he said. "And we keep up with a lot of old friends. It is a lot of work. People don't do it, so you have to do it yourself." I asked who he considered to be his closest friend. He thought for a while and mentioned a couple that they get together with regularly to go museum hopping, to share travel stories and pictures. "There are several people in this play reading group," he said, "that are very close friends." He also feels close to his "only surviving roommate" [from college] who lives in Cambridge, but acknowledged that he didn't see him very often anymore. "Probably our closest friends are here now," he said. Most are people they have met in the years since he retired.

Pete is a great of example of a participant actively finding and maintaining friends. And he was right: keeping up with old friends is a lot of work and many people find it difficult or don't bother. But he and his wife were both predisposed to doing so and particularly enjoyed large gatherings. We're not all that way. Not all of us (or even very many of us) are going to get excited to host twenty people at our house a few times a month. But the point is to understand what kind of connections help us thrive. Are we getting enough of those connections? If not, are there steps we can take in that direction?

THE PATH AHEAD

Listening is a magnetic and strange thing, a creative force. . . . the friends that really listen to us are the ones we move toward. . . . When we are listened to, it creates us, makes us unfold and expand.

Brenda Ueland

Friendships are some of the easiest relationships to neglect. Over and over throughout the lives of Harvard Study participants we see friendships that have deteriorated, for both men and women, because of neglect. Part of what makes friendships wonderful is also what makes them fleeting: they are voluntary. But that doesn't make them any less significant. So you may need to be purposeful about maintaining the friendships you already have, and about creating new friendships.

One of the most common questions people ask us is: *How many friends do I need? Five? Ten? One?*

Unfortunately, we can't answer this question for you! People are just too different. You may feel at your best with two close friends, or you may feel at your best with a whole host of friends that you share different activities with and invite over for large gatherings. Depending on which stage of life you're in, you may find yourself needing different things. You might start looking toward causes and activities that you care about and developing new friends and communities around those. To discover what is best and most fulfilling for you will take some self-reflection. But here are some things to think about regarding the friends in your life:

Friendships can suffer from some of the same things that family relationships suffer from: chronic conflict, boredom, absence of curiosity, failure to pay attention.

Learn to listen to your friends. As Brenda Ueland suggests, listening does as much for the listener as for the person being listened to. Truly absorbing the experience of another person encourages both the listener and the speaker to "unfold," to emerge from our shells, and our lives are often richer for it. We all have sensitive spots in our lives that make navigating the most intimate conversations more difficult, but the rewards are worth the effort. For example, people are often very private about an illness, and would like to be able to share, but worry about burdening their friends. Just showing that you'd like to hear more when they mention a medical concern may be enough to open that door.

Being listened to makes us feel understood, cared for, and *seen*. You may find that simply being there for a friend and listening creates an environment in which you yourself are seen and heard . . . but you have to be brave enough to give your friends something to listen to. It's also often the case in friendships that one person is more likely to listen, and the other more likely to talk. Figure out which one you are; there might be opportunities to balance things out. The strongest friendships flow both ways.

Consider the rifts in your life. Friendships can cause us hurt that we harbor for a long time. But rifts between friends don't have to be permanent.

Sometimes all it takes is a simple *mea culpa*, or an olive branch—a kind text message, an offer to buy lunch, a quick birthday call—to repair a wound from the past. Sometimes we might righteously protect that sense of injury more tenaciously than we ever protected the friendship itself. Letting grudges go can free us from that burden.

Finally, think about your social routines. We often fall into routines with the friends we see most frequently. We talk about the same types of things, the same troubles, over and over. Is there more you would like from a particular friend? Is there more you can give? Perhaps there is more you want to know about that friend or their past. Or something new that the two of you could explore together.

Reading this chapter, you may be thinking that these kinds of efforts are beyond your ability. You might feel lonely, but you also feel set in your ways. Old social habits are hard to change, and we all have certain psychological barriers, like shyness or aversion to groups, that make changing our social circumstances difficult. Maybe you feel it's too late for you.

If this is you, you're not alone. A common refrain among some Harvard Study participants, regardless of gender, is the view that at some point in adult life, it becomes impossible to change the nature of our friendships. Expressions of loneliness in the Study will often be followed by statements like, "I suppose that's just how it is . . ." or "Life just gets too busy for friends . . ." Even in a written response on a formal questionnaire, you can almost hear the resignation in participants' voices.

Andrew Dearing was one of these. Deep down, he just knew that his life would never change. Like many people—perhaps like you—he believed that it was too late.

IT'S TOO LATE FOR ME

Andrew Dearing lived one of the most difficult and lonely lives of any Study participant. As a child, his father was absent, his mother and siblings had to move constantly from one place to another, and he didn't develop any lasting friends. In his early adulthood his struggles with meaningful friendships continued, and he was 34 when he married. His wife was quite critical of Andrew and was averse to most social situations. She didn't want to see anybody, and she didn't want him to see anybody. They never went out, and they rarely had anyone over to visit. His marriage was one of the greatest stresses of his life.

The only thing in life that made him happy was his work. He was a clock repairman, and he enjoyed taking apart old grandfather clocks and cuckoo clocks and making them run again. People always came in with family stories about their clocks, and he felt good about bringing these heirlooms back to life for customers. When asked in his late 50s at what age he planned to retire, he wrote, "I don't know for sure. I have been working since I was eight years old. Work has kept me alive. Retiring sounds and feels like it's the end of the road. So I would like to continue working."

But through most of his adult life, he reported very low levels of happiness and satisfaction. At the age of 45, at a moment of deep despair, Andrew attempted suicide. Twenty years later, he was still struggling. "I've thought of ending it," he wrote in the margins of one questionnaire.

When asked in his mid-60s to describe his closest friends in life and what they had meant to him, Andrew wrote simply, "No one." When asked what he did for fun, he wrote, "I don't do anything. I stay home all the time except to go to work."

When Andrew was 67, his eyesight had deteriorated to the point that he could no longer execute precision work on clocks, and he was forced to retire. Shortly afterward, he went to a therapist for the first time in his life. There he discussed how alone he felt in the world, and how sad he was about having to end his work. He shared that he was having suicidal thoughts. The therapist asked if he'd ever thought of leaving his wife. Andrew hadn't. He felt it would be unkind to her. But the conversation stuck with him, and the next year at the age of 68, although he didn't divorce his wife, he separated from her, and moved into an apartment by himself.

Now, though he was relieved to be free of the constraints of his marriage, Andrew felt lonelier than ever. On a whim, he decided he would start going to the health club near his house and exercise to get his mind off things. He began to go every day, and noticed he was seeing the same people there, day in and day out. One day he said hello to another regular and introduced himself.

Three months later, Andrew knew everyone at the club and had more friends than he'd ever had in his life. Every day he looked forward to his time at the health club, and he began to see some of his friends outside of the club. He discovered that a few of them shared a love for old movies, and they started having get-togethers to screen their favorite films for each other.

A couple of years later, when asked on a Study questionnaire if he ever felt lonely, Andrew wrote, "Yes, often." After all, he was now living alone. But when asked how ideal his life was on a scale from 1 to 7, Andrew circled "7" for "close to ideal." Even though he still felt lonely, his life was so much more fulfilling than it had been that he almost couldn't imagine it getting any better.

Eight years after that, in 2010, Andrew was still close with many of the same friends, had expanded his social circle even further, and expressed great relief that he had changed his life. When he'd been asked years earlier how often he left his home to see others or had people visit him, he'd answered, "Never."

Now, when asked the same question in his 80s, he answered, "Daily."

Because life circumstances vary so much, because people themselves vary so much over time, it's difficult to make a blanket statement about what is and isn't possible in someone's life. But Andrew was one of the most isolated and lonely people in the Study, and he found relief. He changed his routine and connected with others, and in the process extended himself into the world in a way that made him feel valued.

We live in a world that hungers for greater human connection. Sometimes we might feel that we are adrift in life, that we're alone and that we're past the point where we can do anything to change that. Andrew had felt this way. He'd believed that he was long, long past that point. But he was wrong. It wasn't too late. Because the truth is, it's never too late.

Conclusion

IT'S NEVER TOO LATE TO BE HAPPY

Harvard Study Questionnaire, 1983:

> Q: Every investigation alters what is being investigated.
> Over the past few decades what alterations has the Harvard
> Study made in your life?

In 1941 Henry Keane was 14 years old, and healthy. While he lived in a neighborhood defined by poverty, and this deprivation led many of the kids he knew into trouble, Henry had somehow avoided that path. Interested in understanding why, a young researcher from Harvard walked up the three flights of Henry's tenement on a rainy day to talk to Henry and his parents about participating in a cutting-edge research project. Researchers hoped to give him regular physical health check-ups and talk with him about his life periodically for several years to see what they could learn about the lives of young boys in the poorest areas of Boston. Close to five hundred other boys his age from other Boston neighborhoods were also being recruited, most of them from immigrant families like Henry's.

Henry's parents were skeptical, but the researcher seemed trustworthy. They agreed.

A few years before that, Leo DeMarco and John Marsden, both 19-year-old sophomores at Harvard College, made appointments at the Student Health Services office to meet with Arlie Bock, who signed them up for a similar study looking at what made young men thrive. After their first two-hour interviews, he had each of them come back the following week.

"I just can't imagine," John said, "what more you could possibly have to ask me. I never thought I had more than two hours' worth of things to say about myself."

Both of these studies were meant to go on for several years. Maybe ten years, if they could find more funding.

These three boys had their entire lives in front of them. Looking at their intake photos today, Bob and Marc feel a sense of wonder and nostalgia similar to what we might feel looking at the photograph of an old friend. None of the participants could know the challenges they would face, none of them could see where life would take them.

Some of their cohort, boys just like them, died in the coming war. Some died of complications related to alcoholism. Some became rich, some even became famous.

Some lives were happy. Some were not.

Eighty years later we now know that Henry and Leo are in the happy group. They grew into engaged, healthy men, with positive and realistic views of the world. We look at their files—at their lives—and within the normal flow of bad luck and tragedy and hard times, we see some lucky breaks. They fell in love, they adored their children, they found meaning in their communities. They led lives that were largely positive and that they felt grateful for having lived.

John is in the unhappy group. He started life with privileges, including material wealth, and also caught some lucky breaks. He was a brilliant student, went to Harvard, and fulfilled his dream of becoming a successful lawyer. But his mother died when he was 16 and he was also bullied as a child for many years. Over time, he developed a wariness of people and habitually negative ways of coping with the world. He had difficulty connecting with others, and when he encountered challenges, his instinct was to withdraw from the people closest to him. He married twice, and never felt that he was truly loved.

How might we have helped John if we could go back to that day he had his picture taken at age 19? Could we use some of what John helped the Study discover to help him cope with his life? *Here*, we might say to him, *This is the life of someone we studied. He lived it so that you might do it better.*

But many of the most significant findings, naturally, came *after* the participants had already lived much of their lives. So they didn't have the benefit of the research we've presented at the times when it would have helped them most.

That's why we wrote this book: to share with you what we couldn't share with them. Because one thing the large body of research into human flourishing clearly shows—from our longitudinal study and from dozens of others—is that *it doesn't matter how old you are, where you are in the life cycle, whether you are married or not married, introverted or extroverted; everyone can make positive turns in their life.*

John Marsden is a pseudonym. His profession and other identifying details have been changed to protect his identity. The real man behind the name has unfortunately passed away. It's too late for him. But if you're reading this book, it's not too late for you.

LIVING AN EXAMINED LIFE

It has often been asked about the Harvard Study: Did the Study's questions affect how participants lived? Are the data distorted by a kind of psychological Heisenberg effect, where the participants' lives are shaped by the act of self-examination?

This was a question that Arlie Bock and all the subsequent Study directors and researchers have been interested in. On one hand, it's an impossible question to answer. As the saying goes, we can never step into the same river twice: there's no way to know what each participant's life would have been like if they'd not been involved in the Study. The participants themselves, however, had some ideas:

"Sorry, but I don't think it has had any influence," was one typical response.

"Only as a topic of conversation. Sorry!" was another.

John Marsden answered simply: "None."

Joseph Cichy (Chapter Seven) also wrote, "None," and then offered what he believed to be the reason: "I have not had feedback which I can translate into a message for me."

Others, however, acknowledged turning the Study's investigations around, and using them to consider their lives and to open themselves to the possibilities of living differently.

"The Study has caused me to reassess my life every two years," one participant wrote.

Another laid out his entire self-assessment regimen: "It makes me review, challenge present activities, take stock, clarify directions and priorities, and assess my marital relationship, which after thirty-seven years has become so basic a part of life as to be unquestioned."

"Makes me reflect for a bit," Leo DeMarco wrote. "Makes me rejoice in my circumstances; a lovely wife who generally tolerates my foibles. The questions make me aware that there are other lifestyles, other options, other experiences which are *might-have-beens* but weren't."

The fact that participants were affected by the Study's questions is itself a useful lesson for the rest of us. We may not have the Study calling us on the phone and bugging us to answer questions every two years, but we can still take a moment now and then to consider where we are and where we would like to be. It is these moments of stepping back, and looking at our lives, that can help us clear the fog and choose a path forward.

But which path?

We tend to think we know what makes us feel fulfilled, what is good for us, and what is bad for us. No one knows us, we think, quite like we know ourselves. The problem is we're so good at being ourselves, we don't always see that there might be another way.

Recall the wisdom of the Zen master Shunryu Suzuki: "In the beginner's mind there are many possibilities, but in the expert's mind there are few."

Asking honest questions about ourselves is the first step toward recognizing that we may not be experts on our own lives. When we accept this, and we accept that we may not have all the answers, we step into the realm of possibility. And that is a step in the right direction.

IN PURSUIT OF SOMETHING BIGGER

In 2005 we had a luncheon for the inner-city Boston participants, who at that time were in their 70s. There was a table for Southie (South Boston), Roxbury, the West End, the North End, Charlestown, and all the other Boston neighborhoods represented in the Study. Some of the participants even knew each other from school or by virtue of having grown up in the same neighborhoods. Some traveled from across the country and came dressed in their best suits and ties, others just drove to the West End from around the corner, dressed in whatever they happened to be wearing that day. Some brought their wives and their children, many of whom have joined the Study themselves.

Our participants' dedication to the Study has been humbling. Eighty-four percent of our First Generation participants continued their involvement for their entire lives. The typical longitudinal study has a much higher dropout rate and does not come close to covering entire lifetimes. What's more, 68 percent of their children agreed to take part in the Second Generation study—an astonishingly high rate of participation. Even those First Generation participants who have long since passed away made contributions that will affect research for years to come. They've left us with vials of their blood, which in combination with their health and psychological data and historical assessments of Boston neighborhoods are being used to study the long-term health effects of lead and other environmental contaminants. As they approached the end of their lives, some participants even agreed to donate their brains to the Study. Honoring these requests was not easy for their families, who had to go through considerable inconvenience at a time of mourning in order to make sure that the Study could take possession of their loved ones' remains. Thanks to all of this dedication, participants' lives continue to matter, and their legacy will live on.

This has been a mutually life-enhancing project. We, the generations of Harvard Study staff members, have been enlivened by our connection to the participants. In turn, the creativity and commitment of our staff members has enabled hundreds of families to be part of something unique in the history of science. Lewise Gregory, whom we mentioned in Chapter Ten and who worked for the Study for most of its lifespan, is one of the best examples of this. Our participants responded to questionnaires during some of the busiest and most difficult times of their lives not only because they believed in the research, but also because they felt loyal to Lewise and other Study staff. A study that slowly uncovered the value of relationships was itself sustained, in the end, by relationships.

Over the years, these relationships formed a kind of invisible community. Some participants didn't meet anyone else in the Study until very late in their lives and others never knew a single other person who was involved. But they felt a connection to the Study nonetheless. Some participants, wary of self-disclosure, were reluctant in the beginning but continued anyway. Others looked forward to getting calls from the Study and enjoyed the experience of being checked on and listened to. Most, however, were proud to be part of something bigger than themselves. In this way, they thought of the Study as a piece of their own generativity, part of their own mark on the world, and they trusted that eventually their lives would be of use to people they would never meet.

This speaks to a concern that many of us have: *Do I matter?*

Some of us have lived the majority of our lives and find ourselves looking back, others have most of our lives in front of us and are looking forward. For all of us, regardless of age, it helps to remember that this question of mattering, of leaving something for future generations and of being part of something bigger than ourselves, is not just about our personal achievements—it's about what we mean to other people. And it's never too late to start now and leave a mark.

FILLING IN THE GAPS

In the scope of human history, the "science of happiness" is a recent idea. Slowly but surely, science is uncovering useful answers to what makes people thrive across the entire lifespan. New findings, new insights, and new strategies for how to bring happiness research into real life continue to evolve. If you want to keep track of our latest efforts, they can be found at the Lifespan Research Foundation (www.Lifespanresearch.org).

The primary challenge of happiness research comes in the application of insight to actual lives, each of which is highly individual and does not fit neatly into any group template. The findings and ideas we've presented in this book are based on research, but science can't know the turmoil or contradictions you feel in your heart. It can't quantify the stir that you experience when a certain friend calls. It can't know what keeps you up at night, or what you regret, or how you express your love. Science can't say whether you're calling your kids too much or too little, or whether you should reconnect with a particular family member. It can't say if it would be better for you to have a heart-to-heart over a cup of coffee or play a game of basketball or go for a walk with a friend. Those answers can only come through reflection, and figuring out what works for you. For anything in this book to be useful, you will need to tune in to your unique life experience and make its lessons your own.

But here's what science *can* tell you:

Good relationships keep us happier, healthier, and help us live longer.

This is true across the lifespan, and across cultures and contexts, which means it is almost certainly true for you, and for nearly every human being who has ever lived.

THE FOURTH "R"

Few things affect the quality of our lives as much as our connections to others. As we've said many times before, human beings are primarily *social* animals. The implications of that fact may be much vaster than many of us realize.

Basic education is sometimes referred to as the three Rs: reading, writing, and arithmetic. Because early education is meant to prepare students for life, we believe there should be a fourth R in basic education: *relationships.*

Humans are not born with the biological need to read and write, though the skills are now fundamental to society. We are not born with a need to do math, though the modern world would not exist without it. We are, however, born with a need to connect with other people. Because this need for connection is fundamental to a flourishing life, we believe that social fitness should be taught to children and be a central consideration in public policy right alongside exercise, diet, and other health recommendations. Making social fitness central to health education is especially important in the context of rapidly evolving technologies that affect how we communicate and develop relational skills.

There are signs that the world is catching on. There are now hundreds of studies showing that positive relationships have a health benefit, and we've cited many of them in this book. Courses in social and emotional learning (SEL) focus on helping students learn self-awareness, identify and manage emotions, and hone their relationship skills. These programs are being tested in schools all over the world. Across age, race, gender, and class, this research suggests that, compared with students who did not receive this education, students in these programs showed more positive behaviors with peers, had better academic performance, fewer conduct problems, less drug use, and less emotional distress. These programs are a step in the right direction, and their impact shows that this emphasis on relationships pays off. Efforts to bring these same lessons to adults in organizations, workplaces, and community centers are also under way.

ADVERSITY ON THE PATH TO THE GOOD LIFE

We are living in a time of global crisis. Connecting with our fellow human beings takes on new urgency in this context. The Covid-19 pandemic put this need for connection into stark relief. As the disease spread and lockdowns began, many people reached out to solidify the most important relationships in their lives, to boost their sense of connection and security. Then, as the lockdowns stretched from weeks to months and beyond, people began feeling the effects of social isolation in strange and sometimes profound ways. Our bodies and minds, inextricably intertwined, reacted to the stress of isolation. People all over the world began experiencing health impacts as schoolkids lost regular contact with their friends and teachers, workers lost the presence of their workmates, weddings were postponed, friendships sidelined, and those of us who had access to the internet had to settle for connecting through computer screens. Suddenly it became clear that schools, movie theaters, restaurants, and ballparks weren't just about learning, watching movies, eating food, and playing sports. They were about being together.

Global crises will continue to impact our collective well-being. But as we struggle with how to confront these challenges, we must remember that every one of us has only the moment before us, in the place we stand. It is our approach to each unfolding moment and our connections to the individuals we encounter in our lives—family, friends, people in our communities and beyond—that will ultimately serve as a bulwark against whatever crises we confront.

When the Harvard Study participants were kids, they couldn't have envisioned the difficulties they would face, either in the world or in their own lives. Leo DeMarco could not have seen World War II coming. Henry Keane couldn't do anything about the poverty that the Great Depression brought on his family. And we can't foresee exactly what challenges will confront us in the future. But we know they will come.

Thousands of stories from the Harvard Study show us that the good life is not found by providing ourselves with leisure and ease. Rather, it arises from the act of facing inevitable challenges, and from fully inhabiting the moments of our lives. It appears, quietly, as we learn how to love and how to open ourselves to being loved, as we grow from our experiences, and as we stand in solidarity with others through the inevitable string of joys and adversities in every human life.

A FINAL DECISION

How do you move further along on your own path toward a good life? First, by recognizing that the good life is not a destination. It is the path itself, and the people who are walking it with you. As you walk, second by second you can decide to whom and to what you give your attention. Week by week you can prioritize your relationships and choose to be with the people who matter. Year by year you can find purpose and meaning through the lives that you enrich and the relationships that you cultivate. By developing your curiosity and reaching out to others—family, loved ones, coworkers, friends, acquaintances, even strangers—with one thoughtful question at a time, one moment of devoted, authentic attention at a time, you strengthen the foundation of a good life.

We'll make a final suggestion to get you started.

Think about someone, just one person, who is important to you. Someone who may not know how much they really mean to you. It could be your spouse, your significant other, a friend, a coworker, a sibling, a parent, a child, or even a coach or a teacher from your younger days. This person could be sitting beside you as you read or listen to this book, they could be standing over the sink washing dishes, or in another city, another country. Think about where they stand in their lives. What are they struggling with? Think about what they mean to you, what they have done for you in your life. Where would you be without them? Who would you be?

Now think about what you would thank them for if you thought you would never see them again.

And at this moment—right now—turn to them. Call them. Tell them.

ACKNOWLEDGMENTS

This book bears witness to one fundamental truth: We are sustained in a web of relationships that give our life meaning and goodness. We are profoundly grateful to the many people whose kindness and wisdom enabled us to create this work.

The two of us began our friendship and collaboration nearly three decades ago at Massachusetts Mental Health Center, when we were research fellows in the laboratory of Stuart Hauser. His longitudinal study of adolescents introduced us to the riches that can be found in tracking individual lives through time, and Stuart taught us the value of listening to people's stories.

Bob's teacher at Harvard Medical School, George Vaillant, was the third director of the Harvard Study of Adult Development. His insights into adult developmental science have shaped how the world thinks about the human life cycle, and his willingness to entrust this precious longitudinal project to a next generation of researchers was a profoundly generative gift. Of course, we stand on the shoulders of all of the previous directors: Clark Heath, Arlie Bock, and Charles MacArthur, who pioneered the study of the Harvard College student cohort, and Eleanor and Sheldon Glueck, who originated the study of the inner-city Boston cohort. None of this research could happen without funding, and the Harvard Study would not have been possible without support from the

National Institute of Mental Health, the National Institute on Aging, the W. T. Grant Foundation, the Harvard NeuroDiscovery Center, the Fidelity Foundation, the Blum-Kovler Foundation, the Weil Memorial Charitable Foundation, and Ken Bartels and Jane Condon.

Conducting a longitudinal study of this depth requires the dedication and patience of a village. This community included steady shepherds— Lewise Gregory, Eva Milofsky, and Robin Western—who maintained vital connections with our Study participants over decades. And it continues to include a convoy of talented postdoctoral fellows, predoctoral students, undergraduates, and even some high schoolers—too many to name—all of whom have brought curiosity and fresh perspectives that continually enliven our work. Extending the Study to the children of our original participants was only possible with the guidance of a remarkable set of colleagues: Margie Lachman, Kris Preacher, Teresa Seeman, and Ron Spiro. Our colleague Mike Nevarez continues to use his engineer's precision and medical training to oversee the introduction of twenty-first-century biological measures and digital tools in our Second Generation study.

When Bob gave a TEDx talk in 2015 that was widely circulated, it became clear that many people were eager to learn what developmental science can tell us about human thriving. Our friend and colleague John Humphrey had the vision to create and lead the Lifespan Research Foundation (www.lifespanresearch.org), a nonprofit organization with the mission of using the insights of lifespan research to enable people to live healthier lives filled with meaning, connection, and purpose. His death in May of 2022 is a loss we still feel, but we continue to be inspired by his energy and passion for using research to help others. The Foundation team—John, Marianne Doherty, Susan Friedman, Betsy Gillis, Linda Hotchkiss, Mike Nevarez, Connie Steward, and others—has enabled us to take research findings that hide in academic journals and translate them into user-friendly tools for those seeking science-based wisdom about well-being.

The Good Life was the creation of another village: Doug Abrams at Idea Architects had a vision that turned out to be almost exactly what the book became. His belief in the project, and the experience of the Idea

Architects team—particularly Lara Love, Sarah Rainone, and Rachel Neumann—provided clear guidance through the murky terrain of designing and crafting a book about our life's work. Rob Pirro shared with us his deep knowledge of philosophical perspectives on the good life. We were blessed with several generous readers of the manuscript: Cary Crall, Michelle Francl, Kate Petrova, and Jennifer Stone each provided invaluable perspectives and helped sharpen our ideas and writing.

At Simon & Schuster, Jonathan Karp and Bob Bender had the faith to commit to the book at a time of great uncertainty in the world. Their enthusiasm for the project was truly infectious, and it was our good fortune to work with Bob, a seasoned editor whose steady and gentle hand shaped the manuscript with care and wisdom. Johanna Li guided us through the graphic design of the book. We also thank copyeditor Fred Chase. Saliann St-Clair, Jemma McDonagh, Brittany Poulin, and Camilla Ferrier of the Marsh Agency, and Caspian Dennis and Sandy Violette from Abner Stein helped us to bring the book to the wider world through international contracts. And we are grateful to the more than 20 translation publishers who saw the value of bringing the book to people around the globe.

We might not have had the courage to write this book were it not for many people who believed in the project. Tal Ben-Shahar, Arthur Blank, Richard Layard, Vivek Murthy, Laurie Santos, Guy Raz, Jay Shetty, Tim Shriver, and Carol Yu were among those who gave encouragement when we might have gotten cold feet. Our colleagues Angela Duckworth, Eli Finkel, Ramon Florenzano, Peter Fonagy, Julianne Holt-Lunstad, and Dominik Schoebi, who are exemplars of how to bring the insights of scientific research out into the world in accessible and impactful ways, also offered early encouragement.

Mark Hitz was at the center of this project from the beginning. A keen and empathic observer of human experience and a writer of immense skill and subtlety, he learned to dance with us in a world that was completely new to him. He brought an ear for the music of language that you will hear throughout the book. He helped us breathe life into research findings using the stories that he found in reams of Study records. All of this was done with persistence and patience that could only have come from his deep respect for the people who told us their stories. We will always be grateful that Mark turned his talents to this collaboration.

Our greatest debt is to the women and men who participate in the Harvard Study of Adult Development. How do we begin to thank the generations of people who offer their life stories so that the world can gain a richer and deeper understanding of the human condition? In sharing their lives, they give a gift to science and to all of us. They remind us how generous people can be, and how essential it is that we appreciate our shared humanity. We can never repay this debt, but our hope is that, in some small measure, this book pays it forward.

Bob

Whether it's luck or karma, how we find the people who shape our lives is a wonderful mystery. I've benefited from the attention and care of many good mentors. Professor Barbara Rosenkrantz shared her excitement in bringing radical curiosity to musty historical documents. Phil Isenberg, Carolynn Maltas, John Gunderson, and an army of wonderful clinical teachers taught me to bring that same curiosity to the life stories of the people who come to my office seeking relief from mental suffering. Avery Wiseman was a model of the psychoanalyst-scholar, and Tony Kris and George Fishman helped me find the courage to fit clinical practice and empirical research into the same satisfying workdays. Dan Buie and Jil Windsor are rare souls who make people feel truly seen and, in the process, bring out the best in them—including me.

Over the past four decades, I've had the pleasure of working with several hundred young adults as they train to become psychiatrists, and our shared passion for what makes people tick gives me hope for a future where there will always be someone to talk to. Every day I meet with people in my psychotherapy practice, and their courage in sharing their deepest concerns as they face life's difficulties has shown me that the paths to a good and rich life are practically infinite.

Zen meditation is another way in which I explore the experience of being human, and it has been life-altering. My fellow Zen teachers, David Rynick and Michael Fieleke, show me what it means to be present fearlessly for one's life moment after moment. And in giving me dharma transmission, my teacher Melissa Blacker entrusted me with an invaluable and timeless tool for waking up to life that I aspire to bring to everything I encounter.

The Psychiatry Department at Massachusetts General Hospital in Boston continues to be the professional home of my research, teaching, and writing. Maurizio Fava, Jerry Rosenbaum, and John Herman are among the many people who make it exciting and gratifying to be part of this community of clinician-scholars, along with the faculty of the Program in Psychodynamics.

John Makinson brought his droll wisdom and vast publishing experience to this new phase of our fifty-year friendship that never ceases to surprise and delight me. Arthur Blank understood that I needed to write this book long before I knew it—insisting in his gracious and generative way that the insights we'd shared in academic journals should be brought to broader audiences. John Bare had the clear vision of how that could happen.

The family I was born into had everything to do with shaping me and this book. My father, David, was the most curious person I've ever known—endlessly fascinated by the experiences of everyone who crossed his path. My mother, Miriam, demonstrated empathy and connection in everything she did, and my brother, Mark's, mind for family history was a lesson in the value of tracking where we've been in life. For thirty-six years my wife, Jennifer Stone, has been the center of my world—a wise advisor on clinical matters, a careful editor, a willing playmate, and a partner who makes parenting a joyful collaboration. My two sons teach me, tease me, and keep me humble—Daniel with an analytic mind that sometimes makes my jaw drop, and David with playful energy and keen insights that keep refreshing my views of the world.

And of course, my coauthor, Marc Schulz. The story of our friendship is recounted in the book, but it doesn't do justice to three decades of weekly meetings, family visits, and travel to conferences around the world. A typical weekly phone call will range from talking about our kids' challenges at school, to discussing a puzzling clinical situation, to finding the best statistical techniques for analyzing the link between childhood trauma and adult health. Finding a friend whose skills complement and extend my own is probably a once-in-a-lifetime event—and a stroke of good fortune that I never take for granted.

These are the people who remind me every day that a good life can be built with good relationships.

Marc

The Good Life was literally built on the connections we have been lucky enough to have throughout our lives. I grew up with the support of loving parents and grandparents who encouraged me to explore and find joy in the world. My mother is an accomplished photographer who taught me the value of attentively watching and listening to others and the excitement that comes with creative pursuits. She also showed me the pleasure one can get from teaching and mentoring others. My father shared with me his fierce appetite for learning and using knowledge to understand events in our own lives and beyond, as well as the benefits of enjoying life's silly moments. I have also been blessed by incredibly supportive, accepting, and loving stepparents who enriched my life immeasurably.

My grandparents, especially Gladys and Hank, were towering figures for me growing up, and I am grateful for their encouragement and belief in me. My parents and grandparents, each in their own way, have provided valuable models for how to cope with life challenges and how to prioritize relationships. I am also lucky to have three extraordinary siblings who have given me the opportunity to learn about family and life from different perspectives. Julie, Michael, and Suzanne, thank you, for your support and for always being there.

Close friends from childhood and college have shown me both the value of strong connections and the ways they can be sustained across geographical barriers and life circumstances. David Hagen, whom I miss terribly, is an old friend who truly embodied what it meant to be a connector and a life-affirming friend.

I began my formal study of the good life as a college student exploring ideas from sociology, anthropology, political theory, and philosophy at a time when I was really just trying to figure out my own path. Professors Jerry Himmelstein and George Kateb patiently helped me figure out how to unlock mysteries in what I was reading and pushed me to think in new and interesting ways.

Despite my own uncertainty at the time, I decided to study clinical psychology at the University of California at Berkeley. With hindsight, this was one of the great decisions of my life. I began to learn about human thriving and struggling in new ways. Working with clients and figuring out the best ways I could help them with their goals helped me grow in ways for which I am forever grateful. I owe deep thanks to a series of remarkable mentors and clinical supervisors during graduate school and subsequent clinical training. Phil and Carolyn Cowan were critically important mentors who taught me so much about research, clinical work, relationships, and life, including the true value of listening and being curious about the experiences of others. Dick Lazarus was an unusually incisive and creative thinker. He and the Cowans showed me how to research hard-to-quantify, central elements of our lives like emotion and relationships. The wisdom of these and many other teachers permeates the pages of this book.

I have called Bryn Mawr my academic home for more than twenty-five years, and I am enormously privileged to be part of such a vibrant and supportive community of learning. I am grateful to colleagues within and outside the Psychology Department for their support and their commitment to teaching, learning, and research. Kim Cassidy has been a colleague for my entire journey at Bryn Mawr, and I am thankful for her support, encouragement, and friendship throughout these years. Collaborations outside psychology with Michelle Francl, Hank Glassman, and Tim Harte have expanded my thinking and helped inform ideas that we present in this book.

Over the years, I have had the pleasure of teaching and working closely with hundreds of extraordinary students at all levels of training. My connections with students have enriched my life in ways that are hard to describe. I thank all of you, especially the undergraduate and graduate students who have done research with me and helped spark new ideas or sharpen old ones. A special thank you to Kate Petrova, with whom I had the pleasure of working for almost five years and who has helped me refine my thinking about many of the ideas presented in the book. Kate also helped plan the next phase of research for the Harvard Study. Mahek Nirav Shah played an important role in organizing materials and extracting life histories for this book.

Working on this book with Bob has been a true pleasure much like all of the collaborations and adventures we have engaged in over almost three decades. Bob has a combination of smarts, insightfulness, creativity, kindness, and competence that is truly breathtaking. I feel so fortunate that we have been friends and workmates for so long. Ours is a collaboration and friendship through which I have no doubt that we have reached heights together I certainly would not be capable of if I journeyed alone.

My wife and two sons mean the world to me. They give my life layers of meaning and joy that make me feel very, very lucky. Jacob and Sam have always been the best distraction from work the world has ever created. They have grown into kind and thoughtful young men that fill my wife and me with joy and pride. Jacob has a deep interest in the experience of others and in big moral and ethical questions, and I marvel at his gift at communicating complicated ideas. Sam notices patterns and connections that escape others and loves learning about the natural world in ways that are inspiring. My relationships with them and the things they have taught me have made *The Good Life* better.

Joan has been a remarkable companion in life for more than three decades. She has encouraged my pursuits, buoyed my confidence when it wavered, and brought more joy to my life than I deserve. Her kindness, intelligence, and common sense have all helped me focus on what is really important in life. Making a family with Joan has been the best project of my life, and I look forward to navigating together whatever the rest of life has to offer.

NOTES

Chapter 1: What Makes a Good Life?

1 *"There isn't time, so brief is life"*: Samuel Clemens, Mark Twain, wrote this in an August 20, 1886, letter to Clara Spaulding. https://en.wikiquote.org/wiki/Mark_Twain.

1 *In a 2007 survey, millennials were asked:* This survey information comes from Jean M. Twenge and colleagues (2012), "Generational Differences in Young Adults' Life Goals, Concern for Others, and Civic Orientation."

3 *the good life* unfolds, *through time. It is a process:* The psychologist Carl Rogers had a similar idea about the pursuit of a good life being a journey. In 1961, in *On Becoming a Person* (p. 186), he wrote, "The good life is a process not a state of being. It is a direction, not a destination."

10 *the act of* recalling *an event can actually change our memory of it:* Elizabeth Loftus at the University of Washington has done extensive work in this area. For a profile of her, and a summary of her papers on "memory distortion," see Nick Zagorski (2005), "Profile of Elizabeth F. Loftus."

12 *Studies . . . come in two flavors: "cross-sectional" and "longitudinal":* Controlled experiments with random assignment to different conditions are another critical method for understanding human health and behavior. Experiments typically unfold in short passages of time, but they can be used to study some phenomena over longer periods.

14 *most successful prospective longitudinal studies maintain 30 to 70 percent of their participants:* See Kristin Gustavson and colleagues (2012), "Attrition and Generalizability in Longitudinal Studies."

16 *Ananya, from India:* This is the only person in the book outside of the Harvard Study participants whose name is disguised. Like the Study participants, we changed her name to protect her privacy.

20 *The British Cohort Studies:* The Centre for Longitudinal Studies at University College London is the home of four of these five extraordinary studies (https://cls.ucl.ac.uk/cls-studies/). Science journalist Helen Pearson wrote an account of the British Cohort Studies in 2016: *The Life Project.*

20 *The Dunedin Multidisciplinary Health and Development Study:* See Olsson and colleagues (2013), "A 31-Year Longitudinal Study of Child and Adolescent Pathways to Well-Being in Adulthood."

20 *The Kauai Longitudinal Study:* Emmy Werner (1993), "Risk, Resilience, and Recovery."

21 *The Chicago Health, Aging, and Social Relations Study:* John T. Cacioppo and Stephanie Cacioppo (2018), "The Population-Based Longitudinal Chicago Health, Aging, and Social Relations Study."

21 *The Healthy Aging in Neighborhoods of Diversity Across the Life Span:* Tessa K. Novick and colleagues (2021), "Health-Related Social Needs."

21 *the Student Council Study:* The original data and study materials were recently rediscovered and are being maintained by the Harvard Study of Adult Development in preparation for future archiving. The Student Council Study was planned and initiated by Earl Bond, MD, and continued by Rachel Dunaway Cox, PhD. Cox's 1970 book, *Youth into Maturity*, documents the study.

21 *In China, loneliness among older adults has . . . increased:* Ye Luo and Linda J. Waite (2014), "Loneliness and Mortality Among Older Adults in China."

22 *But what we find by looking at the entirety of research:* Research from the Mills Study (R. Helson and colleagues, 2002, "The Growing Evidence for Personality Change in Adulthood") mentioned earlier in this chapter has provided evidence that personality continues to evolve in adulthood.

23 *You can be lonely in a crowd:* John Cacioppo and William Patrick (2008), *Loneliness: Human Nature and the Need for Social Connection.*

23 *The people who were the most satisfied in their relationships at age 50 were the healthiest . . . at age 80:* See 2001 article by George Vaillant and K. Mukamal, "Successful Aging."

23 *Our most happily partnered men and women:* See 2010 paper by Robert J. Waldinger and Marc S. Schulz, "What's Love Got to Do with It?"

23 *A few touchstone examples:* For the HANDLS study, see Tessa K. Novick and colleagues (2021), "Health-Related Social Needs." For the CHASRS findings, see John T. Cacioppo and colleagues (2008), "The Chicago Health, Aging, Social Relations Study." And for the Dunedin findings, see Olsson and colleagues (2013), "A 32-Year Longitudinal Study."

Chapter 2: Why Relationships Matter

27 *"The best ideas aren't hidden in shadowy recesses"*: Richard Farson and Ralph Keyes (2002), *Whoever Makes the Most Mistakes.*

28 *These feelings, big and small . . . feeling of stress:* John T. Cacioppo and colleagues (2014), "Evolutionary Mechanisms for Loneliness."

36 *Researchers at the University of Chicago turned their local train into an affective forecasting experiment:* Nicholas Epley and Juliana Schroeder (2014), "Mistakenly Seeking Solitude."

36 *There is a lot of research . . . human beings are bad at affective forecasting:* See, for example, Timothy D. Wilson and Daniel T. Gilbert (2005), "Affective Forecasting: Knowing What to Want"; and Wilson and Gilbert (2003), "Affective Forecasting."

37 *we pay a lot of attention to potential costs and downplay . . . potential benefits:* Daniel Kahneman and Amos Tversky's seminal research and theory ("Prospect Theory") makes just this point. Kahneman was recognized with a Nobel Prize for this research and theory. See Daniel Kahneman and Amos Tversky (1979), "Prospect Theory: An Analysis of Decision Under Risk." See also A. P. McGraw and colleagues (2010), "Comparing Gains and Losses"; and Gillian M. Sandstrom and Erica J. Boothby (2021) "Why Do People Avoid Talking to Strangers? A Mini Meta-analysis of Predicted Fears and Actual Experiences Talking to a Stranger."

37 *David Foster Wallace used a parable:* Wallace's 2005 commencement address to Kenyon College as quoted in "David Foster Wallace on Life and Work," *Wall Street Journal,* September 19, 2008.

39 *"The life of money-making is one undertaken under compulsion":* Aristotle wrote this in chapter 5 of Nicomachean Ethics in 350 BCE. The quotation can be found online in a translation by W. D. Ross here: http://classics.mit.edu//Aristotle/nicomachaen.html.

39 *"Money has never made man happy, nor will it":* This quote from Benjamin Franklin appears on page 128 of Samuel Austin Allibone's 1880 book, *Prose Quotations from Socrates to Macaulay.*

39 *"Don't make money your goal":* This quote from Maya Angelou was posted on her Facebook page on May 1, 2009.

40 *What We Talk About When We Talk About Money:* Psychologist Abraham Maslow developed a model of human needs, known as "Maslow's Hierarchy of Needs," often represented by a pyramid or triangle divided into five sections, with physiological needs like food, water, and rest at the bottom, "self-actualization" at the very top, and "social belonging" seated directly in the middle. While this model has been criticized for its emphasis on self-actualization, its perspective that the most meaningful areas of life are dependent

upon more basic needs has proven true over many years of research. Any honest answer to the question *What really matters?* must first address physiological needs and safety. We believe that Maslow's third tier, "social belonging," is in the proper place only in that it is at the center of everything.

40 *Angus Deaton and Daniel Kahneman . . . the relationship of money to happiness:* See the 2010 article by Daniel Kahneman and Angus Deaton, "High Income Improves Evaluation of Life but Not Emotional Well-being."

40 *$75,000 per year, which was close to the average family income in the U.S. at the time of the study:* Mean family income in the U.S. in 2010 when Kahneman and Deaton's study was published was $78,180 according to the Federal Reserve Bank of St Louis: https://fred.stlouisfed.org/series/MAFAINUSA646N.

41 *a basic amount of money allows people to . . . have some control over life:* One notable example regarding control at work, which is generally lower in lower-status jobs: the amount of control one has over work schedules and wages was a major predictor of health disparities in the British Whitehall Longitudinal Studies. Workers with less control were sicker. See the 1997 paper by Michael G. Marmot and colleagues, "Contribution of Job Control and Other Risk Factors to Social Variations in Coronary Heart Disease Incidence." See also Hans Bosma and colleagues (1997), "Low Job Control and Risk of Coronary Heart Disease in Whitehall II (Prospective Cohort) Study."

41 *cultures that vary in wealth:* One notable study by Matthew Killingsworth challenges this conclusion. Reported well-being in this study continues to rise when income surpasses $75,000, but to a substantially narrower degree with each increase. See Killingsworth (2021) and Kieran Healy (2021).

41 *"More money does not necessarily buy more happiness . . . emotional pain.":* See Kahneman and Deaton (2010).

42 *"badges of ability":* Richard Sennett and Jonathan Cobb (1972), *The Hidden Injuries of Class.*

42 *the more we compare ourselves to others . . . the less happy we are:* See the 2015 paper by Philippe Verduyn and colleagues, "Passive Facebook Usage Undermines Affective Well-being: Experimental and Longitudinal Evidence." Also see Judith B. White and colleagues (2006), "Frequent Social Comparisons and Destructive Emotions and Behaviors: The Dark Side of Social Comparisons."

45 *Reinhold Niebuhr's "Serenity Prayer":* A version of this prayer is now commonly used in Alcoholics Anonymous and other twelve-step programs.

46 *startling and influential paper published in the journal* Science: See the article by James S. House and colleagues (1988), "Social Relationships and Health."

46 *Blacks had a higher risk of dying . . . though that difference was relatively small:* These disparities continue to exist. In the United States, whites live 3.6 years

longer than Blacks (Max Roberts, Eric N. Reither, and Sojoung Lim, 2020, "Contributors to the Black-White Life Expectancy Gap in Washington D.C."). In the U.S., for individuals born in 2016, life expectancy overall is 78.7. In Finland, life expectancy is 81.4 These data come from: https://data.worldbank.org/ indicator/SP.DYN.LE00.FE.IN?end=2019&locations=FI&start=2001.

47 *another much larger study cemented the connection between relationships and risk of mortality:* Julianne Holt-Lunstad and colleagues (2010), "Social Relationships and Mortality: A Meta-analytic Review."

47 *the leading cause of preventable death:* U.S. Department of Health and Human Services, Centers for Disease Control and Prevention, National Center for Chronic Disease Prevention and Health Promotion, Office on Smoking and Health: "The Health Consequences of Smoking—50 Years of Progress: A Report of the Surgeon General." Atlanta: 2014. https://www.cdc.gov/tobacco /data_statistics/sgr/50th-anniversary/index.htm

47 *study after study . . . continues to reinforce the connection between good relationships and health:* In 2015, Julianne Holt-Lunstad and colleagues published another meta-analysis showing that social isolation and loneliness were both associated with increased likelihood of mortality. See Holt-Lunstad and colleagues (2015), "Loneliness and Social Isolation as Risk Factors for Mortality: A Meta-analytic Review."

47 *regardless of a person's location, age, ethnicity, or background:* Three research examples to illustrate the diversity of samples showing the association of social connections and health (both physical and psychological):

In the Healthy Aging in Neighborhoods of Diversity Across the Life Span (HANDLS) study in Baltimore with a cohort of 3,720 Black and White adults (aged 35–64), participants that reported receiving more social support also reported less depression. Novick and colleagues (2021), "Health Related Social Needs."

In the birth cohort study based in Dunedin, New Zealand, social connections in adolescence predicted well-being in adulthood better than academic achievement. Olsson and colleagues (2013), "A 32-Year Longitudinal Study."

In the Chicago Health, Aging, and Social Relations Study (CHASRS), a representative study of Chicago residents, those who were in satisfying relationships reported higher levels of happiness. John Cacioppo and colleagues (2018), "The Population-Based Longitudinal Chicago Health, Aging, and Social Relations Study."

49 *Our actions . . . account for about 40 percent of our happiness:* This estimate comes from interesting work done by Sonja Lyubomirsky and colleagues in 2005, "Pursuing Happiness: The Architecture of Sustainable Change."

50 *David Foster Wallace, in his Kenyon commencement:* Wallace (2018), "David Foster Wallace on Life and Work."

52 *"Love by its very nature . . . is unworldly":* Hannah Arendt (1958), *The Human Condition.*

Chapter 3: Relationships on the Winding Road of Life

54 *"Our destiny is frequently met in the very paths we take to avoid it":* From La Fontaine's fable "The Horoscope." This is a common translation of the French. It is also translated as "Fearing the fate that one would skirt, it / often befalls that, rather than avert it, / One takes the path that leads to it directly." La Fontaine, *The Complete Fables,* p. 209.

59 *The Greeks had various versions . . . grammar school:* For a description of the Greeks' versions of life stages, see R. Larry Overstreet (2009), "The Greek Concept of the 'Seven Stages of Life' and Its New Testament Significance." For the origin of Shakespeare's life stages, see T. W. Baldwin (1944), *William Shakespeare's Small Latine and Lesse Greeke.*

59 *Islamic teachings:* For a summary of Islam's seven stages of existence, see https://www.pressreader.com/nigeria/thisday/20201204/281977495192204.

59 *Buddhist teachings illustrate the ten stages along the path to enlightenment:* See Pia Tan (2004), "The Taming of the Bull."

59 *Hinduism identifies four stages of life:* See Pradeep Chakkarath (2013), "Indian Thoughts on Psychological Human Development."

60 *Erik and Joan Erikson, framed adult development as a series of key challenges:* These ideas were introduced in a series of publications including the following books: Erik Erikson (1950), *Childhood and Society;* Erik Erikson (1959), *Identity and The Life Cycle;* and Erik Erikson and Joan M. Erikson (1997), *The Life Cycle Completed: Extended Version.*

60 *Bernice Neugarten . . . timing of the events in our lives:* See the 1976 article by Bernice Neugarten, "Adaptation and the Life Cycle."

60 *Many who identify as LGBTQ+ experience themselves as "off-time":* See Sara Jaffe (2018), "Queer Time."

61 *vast literature available on the human life cycle:* In addition to the work by Joan and Erik Erikson and by Bernice Neugarten cited above, here is a small selection of books and articles about the life cycle: Gail Sheehy (1996), *New Passages: Mapping Your Life Across Time;* David Levinson (1996), *The Seasons of a Woman's Life;* George Vaillant (2002), *Aging Well;* and Paul B. Baltes (1997), "On the Incomplete Architecture of Human Ontogeny."

62 *Richard Bromfield captured the feeling of loving a teenager well:* Bromfield metaphor of tightropes and the quote that follows comes from his 1992 book, *Playing for Real,* pp. 180–81.

63 *Anthony Wolf's popular parenting book:* See Wolf's 2002 book, *Get Out of My Life, but First Could You Drive Me and Cheryl to the Mall?*

64 *advantages for adolescents who become more autonomous:* See the 1994 article by Joseph Allen and colleagues, "Longitudinal Assessment of Autonomy and Relatedness in Adolescent-Family Interactions as Predictors of Adolescent Ego Development and Self-Esteem."

64 *One participant in the Student Council Study:* This quotation was included in Rachel Dunaway Cox's 1970 book about the Student Council Study, *Youth into Maturity*, p. 231.

64 *that standard joke of Mark Twain's:* This participant is referring to a story, often attributed to Mark Twain, that goes like this: "When I was a boy of fourteen, my father was so ignorant I could hardly stand to have the old man around. But when I got to be twenty-one, I was astonished at how much he had learned in seven years."

71 *Jeffrey Arnett has labeled:* Jeffrey Arnett (2000), "Emerging Adulthood: A Theory of Development from the Late Teens Through the Twenties."

71 *In 2015, one third of U.S. adults aged 18–34 lived with their parents . . . 2.2 million young adults, were neither attending school nor working:* Jonathan Vespa (2017), "The Changing Economics and Demographics of Young Adulthood, 1975–2016."

78 *In a study done in 2003 . . . participants . . . were shown two advertisements:* Helene H. Fung and Laura L. Carstensen (2003), "Sending Memorable Messages to the Old: Age Differences in Preferences and Memory for Advertisements."

78 *If we think we have less time, we try to appreciate the present:* These ideas have been articulated by Laura Carstensen as part of her Socioemotional Selectivity Theory, and in her research she has produced much of the evidence that supports them. See, for example, Laura Carstensen and colleagues (1999), "Taking Time Seriously: A Theory of Socioemotional Selectivity." Also: Carstensen (2006), "The Influence of a Sense of Time on Human Development."

79 *human beings are never so happy as in the late years of their lives:* See Carstensen (1999), "Taking Time Seriously."

81 *it's these unexpected turns . . . that most define a person's life:* See Albert Bandura (1982), "The Psychology of Chance Encounters and Life Paths."

82 *This echoes findings from . . . the Dunedin Study:* See the article by A. Caspi and T. E. Moffitt (1995), "The Continuity of Maladaptive Behavior: From Description to Understanding in the Study of Antisocial Behavior."

Chapter 4: Social Fitness: Keeping Your Relationships in Good Shape

86 *"A sad soul can kill you quicker":* This quote comes from Steinbeck's 1962 book, *Travels with Charley: In Search of America*, p. 38.

87 *Janice Kiecolt-Glaser, was investigating psychological stress:* Kiecolt-Glaser is one of the world's foremost experts on the effect of stress on the immune system. She discusses her research and her personal experience with caregiving stress in a 2016 WexMed talk found here: https://www.youtube.com/watch?v=hjUW 2YClOYM. The research on caregivers and wound healing is published in a 1995 article by Kiecolt-Glaser and colleagues, "Slowing of Wound Healing by Psychological Stress."

92 *When you're lonely, it hurts:* Two scholarly reviews of the impact of loneliness are those by Louise Hawkley and John Cacioppo in 2010, "Loneliness Matters: A Theoretical and Empirical Review of Consequences and Mechanisms," and by Cacioppo and Cacioppo in 2012, "The Phenotype of Loneliness." John Cacioppo and William Patrick (2008) have written a book about loneliness for a more general audience—*Loneliness: Human Nature and the Need for Social Connection*—that summarizes relevant research.

92 *Loneliness is associated with:*

Suppression of the immune system: S. D. Pressman and colleagues (2005), "Loneliness, Social Network Size, and Immune Response to Influenza Vaccination in College Freshmen."

Less effective sleep: Sarah C. Griffin, and colleagues (2020), "Loneliness and Sleep: A Systematic Review and Meta-analysis."

Diminished brain function: Aparna Shankar and colleagues (2013), "Social Isolation and Loneliness: Relationships with Cognitive Function During 4 Years of Follow-up in the English Longitudinal Study of Ageing."

92 *loneliness is twice as unhealthy as obesity:* Holt-Lunstad and colleagues (2010), "Social Relationships and Mortality Risk: A Meta-analytic Review."

92 *chronic loneliness increases a person's odds of death . . . 26 percent:* Holt-Lunstad and colleagues (2015), "Loneliness and Social Isolation as Risk Factors for Mortality: A Meta-Analytic Review."

92 *study in the U.K. . . . connections between loneliness and poorer health . . . in young adults:* Timothy Matthews and colleagues (2019), "Lonely Young Adults in Modern Britain: Findings from an Epidemiological Cohort Study."

93 *In a study conducted online . . . one out of every three people . . . feel lonely:* This study, known as the BBC Loneliness Experiment, is summarized by Claudia Hammond, "Who Feels Lonely? The Results of the World's Largest Loneliness Study," BBC Radio 4, May 2018, https://www.bbc.co.uk/programmes/articles /2yzhfv4DvqVp5nZyxBD8G23/who-feels-lonely-the-results-of-the-world-s -largest-loneliness-study. A scholarly article on this study's key findings can be

found here: Manuela Barreto and colleagues (2021), "Loneliness Around the World: Age, Gender, and Cultural Differences in Loneliness." The findings from this study also suggest that loneliness is more prevalent in societies with more individualistic (rather than collectivistic) values and that men are more likely to experience loneliness. These findings are summarized in a 2018 article by Matthews and colleagues. It is important, of course, to note that these correlational findings could also indicate that poorer coping strategies, mental health problems, and risky physical health behaviors contribute to loneliness. It is likely that causal processes operate in both directions.

93 *the economic cost of this loneliness:* Karen Jeffrey and colleagues (2017), "The Cost of Loneliness to UK Employers."

93 *In Japan, 32 percent of adults . . . expected to feel lonely:* IPSOS (March 2020), "2020 Predictions, Perceptions and Expectations," p. 39.

93 *In the United States, a 2018 study suggested . . . moderate to high levels of loneliness:* Ellen Lee and colleagues (2019), "High Prevalence and Adverse Health Effects of Loneliness in Community-Dwelling Adults Across the Lifespan: Role of Wisdom as a Protective Factor."

93 *In 2020 it was estimated that 162,000 deaths . . . social isolation:* Dilip Jeste and colleagues (2020), "Battling the Modern Behavioral Epidemic of Loneliness: Suggestions for Research and Interventions."

94 *When we feel isolated, our bodies . . . help us survive that isolation:* A summary of evolutionary influences to be social can be found in John Cacioppo and colleagues (2014), "Evolutionary Mechanisms for Loneliness."

95 *How does this add up for the coming years?:* An effective dramatization of this calculation can be found in a 2018 advertisement for a Spanish liqueur: "Ruavieja Commercial 2018 (English subs): #WeHaveToSeeMoreOfEachOther," Ruavieja, November 20, 2018.

96 *average American spent . . . eleven hours every day interacting with media:* Nielsen Report (2018), "Q1 2018 Total Audience Report."

97 *In 2008 we telephoned the wives and husbands of Harvard Study couples:* See Waldinger and Schulz (2010), "What's Love Got to Do with It? Social Functioning, Perceived Health, and Daily Happiness in Married Octogenarians."

106 *You can't make old friends:* "You Can't Make Old Friends," track 1, on Kenny Rogers, *You Can't Make Old Friends*, Warner Music Nashville, 2013.

106 *The proportion of people . . . who never marry has increased:* These figures come from a report by Wendy Wang (2020) that uses U.S. Census and national survey data: "More Than One-Third of Prime-Age Americans Have Never Married."

108 *field of research that studies human motivation:* For a discussion of this research, see Kou Murayama (2018), "The Science of Motivation."

110 *"We are self-centered and selfish . . . this will take time"*: The Dalai Lama at the American Enterprise Institute conference, "Economics, Happiness, and the Search for a Better Life," February 2014.

110 *Being generous . . . make us more likely to help others in the future*: Soyoung Q. Park and colleagues (2017), "A Neural Link Between Generosity and Happiness."

112 *A positive, trusting relationship with a spouse can make a . . . person feel more secure*: For relevant research, see work by Nickola Overall and Jeffrey Simpson (2014), "Attachment and Dyadic Regulation Processes"; Deborah Cohen and colleagues (1992), "Working Models of Childhood Attachment and Couple Relationships"; and M. Kumashiro and B. Arriaga (2020), "Attachment Security Enhancement Model: Bolstering Attachment Security Through Close Relationships."

113 *Every man I meet is my master in some point*: Ralph Waldo Emerson (1876), *Letters and Social Aims*, p. 280.

Chapter 5: Attention to Relationships: Your Best Investment

117 *"The only gift is a portion of thyself"*: This quotation comes from Emerson's essay on gifts and can be found in the Great Books online version created by Bartleby.com of the Harvard Classics edition of *Essays and English Traits by Emerson* (1844) on p. 2.

117 *Harvard Study Second Generation Questionnaire, 2015*: These questions are taken from the Short Form of the Five Facets of Mindfulness Questionnaire (FFMQ-SF) created by Ernst Thomas Bohmeijer and colleagues (2011), "Psychometric Properties of the Five-Facet Mindfulness Questionnaire in Depressed Adults and Development of a Short Form."

119 *"Attention is the rarest"*: See Simone Weil, *Gravity and Grace* (2002).

119 *"Attention . . . is the most basic form of love"*: See John Tarrant, *The Light Inside the Dark*, 1998.

121 *those of us who feel time-poor are more stressed and less healthy*: Ashley V. Whillans and colleagues (2017), "Buying Time Promotes Happiness." See also an article intended for a more general audience about time pressure and unhappiness by Ashley Whillans, (2019), "Time Poor and Unhappy."

121 *Globally, average work hours have declined*: Charlie Giattino and colleagues (2013), "Working Hours." See also Derek Thompson (2014), "The Myth That Americans Are Busier Than Ever."

121 *caveats about who is working more, who is working less*: Magali Rheault (2011), "In U.S., 3 in 10 Working Adults Are Strapped for Time."

121 *we still feel that our time is stretched to the max*: For more on the subjective nature of our experience of free time, see M. A. Sharif and colleagues (2021),

"Having Too Little or Too Much Time Is Linked to Lower Subjective Well-being." They found that the amount of free time we have is not the only important factor: *what we do* with that time is also very important.

122 *In a 2010 study, Matthew Killingsworth and Daniel Gilbert:* See Matthew Killingsworth and Daniel T. Gilbert (2010), "A Wandering Mind Is an Unhappy Mind."

123 *Switching from one task to another takes energy and a measurable amount of time:* Timothy J. Buschman and colleagues (2011), "Neural Substrates of Cognitive Capacity Limitations."

123 *"continuous partial attention":* James Fallows (2013), "Linda Stone on Maintaining Focus in a Maddeningly Distractive World."

126 *Attention . . . equally valuable no matter what era a person lives in:* For a discussion of past worries about technological progress, see A. Orben (2020), "The Sisyphean Cycle of Technology Panics."

127 *when social media is used to sustain relationships . . . connectedness and belonging:* Philippe Verduyn and colleagues (2017), "Do Social Network Sites Enhance or Undermine Subjective Well-being? A Critical Review."

128 *As data from our own Harvard Study (and many others) . . . how they developed as children:* Two examples from our own research showing links between childhood relationship experiences and later relationship functioning: Robert J. Waldinger and Marc S. Schulz (2016), "The Long Reach of Nurturing Family Environments: Links with Midlife Emotion-Regulatory Styles and Late-Life Security in Intimate Relationships"; and Sarah W. Whitton and colleagues (2008), "Prospective Associations from Family-of-Origin Interactions to Adult Marital Interactions and Relationship Adjustment."

128 *we can't assume that online spaces . . . skills they can also develop online:* This is a rapidly expanding area of research. See, for example, additional relevant work by Kate Petrova and Marc Schulz (2022), "Emotional Experiences in Digitally Mediated and In-Person Interactions: An Experience-Sampling Study"; Tatiana A. Vlahovic and colleagues (2012), "Effects of Duration and Laughter on Subjective Happiness Within Different Modes of Communication"; Donghee Y. Wohn and Robert LaRose (2014), "Effects of Loneliness and Differential Usage of Facebook on College Adjustment of First-Year Students"; and Verduyn and colleagues (2017), "Do Social Network Sites Enhance or Undermine Subjective Well-being? A Critical Review."

129 *In nursing homes where social media . . . social isolation . . . official cause of death:* Christopher Magan (2020), "Isolated During the Pandemic Seniors Are Dying of Loneliness and Their Families Are Demanding Help."

129 *Despite our virtual connectedness . . . loneliness worsened:* For discussions of how the Covid pandemic affected loneliness and mental health, see Tzung-Jeng

Hwang and colleagues (2020), "Loneliness and Social Isolation During the COVID-19 Pandemic"; Mark E. Czeisler and colleagues (2020), "Mental Health, Substance Use, and Suicidal Ideation During the COVID-19 Pandemic"; William D. S. Killgore and colleagues (2020), "Loneliness: A Signature Mental Health Concern in the Era of COVID-19"; and Christopher J. Cronin and William N. Evans (2021), "Excess Mortality from COVID and Non-COVID Causes in Minority Populations." Despite the broad effects of lockdowns, trends in loneliness across the entire pandemic are complicated and studies are not fully consistent. For example, one prominent review suggests that loneliness did not increase globally (on average) during the first year of the pandemic: L. Aknin and colleagues (2021), "Mental Health During the First Year of the COVID-19 Pandemic: A Review and Recommendations for Moving Forward."

130 *How an individual uses these platforms matters:* For a discussion of this research, see Verduyn and colleagues (2015), "Passive Facebook Usage Undermines Affective Well-being: Experimental and Longitudinal Evidence"; and also Ethan Kross and colleagues (2013), "Facebook Use Predicts Declines in Subjective Well-Being in Young Adults."

130 *those who use Facebook passively:* P. Verduyn and colleagues (2015), "Passive Facebook Usage Undermines Affective Well-being: Experimental and Longitudinal Evidence."

130 *A similar conclusion was reached in a study in Norway:* Michael Birkjaer and Micah Kaats (2019), "Does Social Media Really Pose a Threat to Young People's Well-being?"

130 *those who compare themselves to others . . . are less happy:* See relevant work by Verduyn and colleagues (2015), "Passive Facebook Usage Undermines Affective Well-being: Experimental and Longitudinal Evidence"; and research by Ursula Oberst and colleagues (2015) studying over 1,400 adolescents in Latin America: "Negative Consequences from Heavy Social Networking in Adolescents: The Mediating Role of Fear of Missing Out."

131 *Are your online habits affecting them?:* Elyssa M. Barrick and colleagues (2020), "The Unexpected Social Consequences of Diverting Attention to Our Phones."

132 *The present moment is the only time over which we have dominion:* This quote appears on page 74 of Thich Nhat Hanh's (2016) book, *The Miracle of Mindfulness.*

132 *a large number of medical schools now offer mindfulness training:* Laura Buchholz (2015), "Exploring the Promise of Mindfulness as Medicine."

132 *"the awareness that emerges . . . things as they are":* J. M. Williams and colleagues (2007), *The Mindful Way Through Depression.*

132 *Even the U.S. military is invested in mindfulness:* See Anthony P. Zanesco and colleagues (2019), "Mindfulness Training as Cognitive Training in High-Demand

Cohorts: An Initial Study in Elite Military Servicemembers." See also Amishi Jha and colleagues (2019), "Deploying Mindfulness to Gain Cognitive Advantage: Considerations for Military Effectiveness and Well-being."

134 *designed a study to help work this out . . . diverse backgrounds:* In this study (Cohen and colleagues, 2012), half of the couples were formally married and the others were in long-term committed relationships. Thirty-one percent had a high school education or less, 29 percent were people of color. See Shiri Cohen and colleagues (2012), "Eye of the Beholder: The Individual and Dyadic Contributions of Empathic Accuracy and Perceived Empathic Effort to Relationship Satisfaction."

Chapter 6: Facing the Music: Adapting to Challenges in Your Relationships

140 *"There is a crack, a crack in everything":* This lyric is from Leonard Cohen, the musician and poet. It can be found on Cohen's (1992) *Anthem*, track 5, on Leonard Cohen, *The Future* album. Cohen's lyric has many precursors, and probably originates with Ralph Waldo Emerson: "There is a crack in every thing God has made," from *Essays*, p. 88.

141 *"There are two pillars of happiness . . . does not push love away":* George Vaillant, *Triumphs of Experience*, p. 50.

146 *Many studies have shown that when we avoid confronting challenges . . . it can get worse:* Two examples of relevant research are Shelly L. Gable (2006), "Approach and Avoidance Social Motives and Goals"; and E. A. Impett and colleagues (2010), "Moving Toward More Perfect Unions."

146 *we used data from the Harvard Study and asked . . . face difficulties directly:* We describe this research in Waldinger and Schulz (2010), "Facing the Music or Burying our Heads in the Sand," along with other relevant research.

147 *there are advantages to being flexible:* Richard S. Lazarus (1991), *Emotion and Adaptation*, provided a compelling and influential argument that all efforts at responding to challenges must be matched to the demands of the situation. George Bonanno's research and ideas have also spoken eloquently to the advantages of responding to challenges in flexible ways. See, for example, Bonanno and Burton (2013) and Bonanno and colleagues (2004). Building on Lazarus's and Bonanno's ideas, we (Dworkin and colleagues, 2019) have provided evidence linking flexible coping when discussing relationship challenges with relationship satisfaction.

148 *the connection between how we perceive events and how we feel about them:* For a more thorough discussion of this idea, see Lazarus (1991) and Moors and colleagues (2013).

148 *"Men are disturbed not by events, but by the views they take of them":* This quotation from Epictetus was written in AD 135 in the *Enchiridion*. Elizabeth Carter

(http://classics.mit.edu/Epictetus/epicench.html) offers a slightly different translation: "Men are disturbed, not by things, but by the principles and notions which they form concerning things."

148   *"Monks," the Buddha said:* This quote is attributed to the Buddhist scripture Samyutta Nikaya, in Anne Bancroft's 2017 (p. 7) *The Wisdom of the Buddha: Heart Teachings in His Own Words.*

149   *The W.I.S.E.R Model of Reacting:* The model we present builds on existing models of emotion and coping with challenges including important work by Lazarus and Folkman (1984) and Crick and Dodge (1994).

152   *Emotion is usually a sign that there is something important going on:* This idea comes from several influential theories of emotion, including Lazarus's (1991) seminal work. See also Schulz and Lazarus (2012) for a summary of these ideas.

159   *"The world we live in":* See Shohaku Okumura, *Realizing Genjokoan: The Key to Dogen's Shobogenzo.*

160   *self-distanced reflection can shed new light on old stories:* The benefits of self-distancing have been explored in a number of research studies by Ethan Kross and Ozlem Aduk. See, for example, Kross's (2021) book, *Chatter,* and a summary of relevant research in Kross, Ayduk, and Mischel (2005).

160   *"In the beginner's mind there are many possibilities":* This quote comes from Shunryu Suzuki's 2010 book, *Zen Mind, Beginner's Mind* (p. 1).

161   *The men who fought in the war talked about the bonds they formed:* See 2017 article by Michael Nevarez, Hannah Yee, and Robert Waldinger.

161   *many talked about how important it was to be able to share at least part of their experiences:* See thesis work by Someshwar (2018).

Chapter 7: The Person Beside You: How Intimate Relationships Shape Our Lives

165   *"When we were children":* Madeleine L'Engle, *Walking on Water: Reflections on Faith and Art* (New York: Convergent, 1980), pp. 182–83.

165   *In Plato's* Symposium, *Aristophanes gives a speech:* Plato, *The Symposium,* trans. Christopher Gill (London: Penguin, 1999), pp. 22–24.

166   *the variety of committed relationships is increasing:* These figures are drawn from Joseph Chamie (2021), "The End of Marriage in America?" and Kim Parker and colleagues (2019), "Marriage and Cohabitation in the U.S."

167   *We talked of castles and kings, of cabbages:* It seems James and Maryanne shared an affinity for Lewis Carroll:

"The time has come," the Walrus said,
"To talk of many things:
Of shoes—and ships—and sealing wax—

Of cabbages—and kings—
And why the sea is boiling hot—
And whether pigs have wings."

—"The Walrus and the Carpenter"

Lewis Carroll, *Through the Looking-Glass, and What Alice Found There*, pp. 73–74.

174 *when a securely attached child seeks her caregiver . . . psychological benefits:* For relevant research, see studies by Hills-Soderlund and colleagues (2008), Spangler and colleagues (1998), and Order and colleagues (2020)

175 *Study participants' relationships were affecting their bodies in real time:* James Coan presented this research in a 2013 TEDx Talk, "Why We Hold Hands," in Charlottesville, Virginia. This research is reported in Coan and Colleagues (2006).

175 *The mere thought of a person who is important to us can generate chemicals . . . other body systems:* Research supporting this conclusion comes from a variety of sources including basic research linking thinking to emotions and emotional arousal (e.g., Smith, 1989). Also see work by Krause and colleagues (2016) linking physiological reactions in mothers to thinking about individuals in interpersonal contexts.

176 *emotions are a signal that there are matters of significance to us at play:* See Lazarus (1991).

177 *We investigated the link between emotion and relationship stability:* Research summarized in Waldinger and colleagues (2004).

177 *The fact that raters with no special knowledge of psychology . . . most adults have a facility to accurately read emotions:* In this study, we also compared combined aggregates of our "naive" raters to expert emotion coders and found a very high correspondence between the ratings from these two sources.

178 *A Fear of Differences:* Most of the relevant research and thinking about the role of differences in causing strong emotions in couples comes from work on couples therapy. See, for example, work by Sue Johnson (2013), Daniel Wile (2008), and Schulz, Cowan, and Cowan (2006).

187 *a key lesson of the Harvard Study . . . relationships (and especially intimate relationships) play a crucial role in how satisfied we are at any particular moment in life:* For a discussion of the connection between relationship satisfaction and overall satisfaction in life over time, see McAdams and colleagues (2012) article from the longitudinal study, the British Household Panel Survey.

187 *Life changes of all kinds can cause stress in our intimate partnerships. Even positive changes:* In 1967, Thomas Holmes and Richard Rahe developed a scale to measure the stress associated with life changes. It included events like getting

married, starting a new job, becoming pregnant, experiencing the death of a close friend, and retirement. They gave each event a score of "life change units" from 0–100, and they found that people with higher total life change scores had more physical illness. This scale has been used across many cultures and in a number of different populations, and it's proven useful over the years. The remarkable thing is that the scale is not based on how "negative" or "positive" an event is, but rather on the amount of change it causes.

188 *Many studies, including our own, show that there is often a decline in relationship satisfaction after the birth of a child:* See, for example, Schulz, Cowan, and Cowan (2006). .

192 *There is no remedy for love but to love more:* This quote comes from Thoreau's Journal I, page 88 (July 25, 1839).

194 *technique that shares much in common with mindfulness . . . research showing its utility:* See, for example, Kross (2021) and Kross and Ayduk (2017). For research connecting self-distancing and mindfulness, see Petrova and colleagues (2021).

Chapter 8: Family Matters

196 *"Call it a clan":* This quotation comes from Jane Howard's 1998 book, *Families* (p. 234).

197 *Lowell Street (now Lomasney Way):* See Levesque, "The West End Through Time." Many of our participants' neighborhoods in the West End and other areas of Boston were bulldozed during the period of urban renewal that began in the 1950s, and no longer resemble the places they once were. See the following for a good description of changes in the West End across time: http://web.mit.edu/aml2010/www/throughtime.html.

198 *ongoing debate in the field of psychology. Some believe that early family experience determines who we become:* Sigmund Freud and many of his psychoanalytic followers famously emphasized the role of early childhood experiences in shaping adult personality and functioning. A 1998 book by Judith Rich Harris (*The Nurture Assumption: Why Children Turn out the Way They Do*) ignited a public debate about the degree to which early childhood environments shape later functioning by claiming that most of this connection between early childhood environments and later functioning can be accounted for by genetic influences. Advocates on both sides of this issue continue to debate this issue.

201 *"No man is an island":* This quotation from John Donne can be found on pp. 108–9 of *Devotions Upon Emergent Occasions: Together with Death's Duel.*

201 *In ancient China, the idea of family . . . this model remains strong in China today:* See, for example, Huang and Gove (2012).

202 *"Ballroom culture":* Marlon M. Bailey, *Butch Queens Up in Pumps.*

202 *"In general . . . society at large"*: Marlon M. Bailey, *Butch Queens Up in Pumps*, p. 5.

203 *Regardless of our current lives, we still carry the ghosts of our childhoods:* Selma Fraiberg, an American psychoanalyst and social worker, wrote an influential (1975) article, entitled "Ghosts in the Nursery," about the influence of childhood legacies.

205 *In 1955, a developmental psychologist named Emmy Werner:* Emmy Werner and Ruth S. Smith summarize this research in two books, *Overcoming the Odds: High Risk Children from Birth to Adulthood* (1992); and *Journeys from Childhood to Midlife: Risk, Resilience, and Recovery* (2001).

205 *"[The participants] were children and grandchildren of immigrants . . . a small group of Anglo-Saxon Caucasians"*: Emmy E. Werner and Ruth S. Smith, "An Epidemiologic Perspective on Some Antecedents and Consequences of Childhood Mental Health Problems and Learning Disabilities (A Report from the Kauai Longitudinal Study)," p. 293.

205 *Werner didn't select just a few participants . . . study lasted for over thirty years:* Study summarized in Werner (1993).

205 *One third of all children who had adverse childhoods . . . well-adjusted adults:* Werner and Smith (1979).

206 *Harvard Study participants who were able to acknowledge challenges . . . similar ability to elicit support from others:* Evidence for the benefits associated with acknowledging challenges and talking about them is provided in Waldinger and Schulz (2016).

221 *Any excuse to gather the family together . . . lower rates of substance abuse, teen pregnancy, and depression:* These findings are summarized in Anne Fishel (2016), "Harnessing the Power of Family Dinners to Create Change in Family Therapy."

221 *adults in the U.S. eating about half of their meals alone:* Reported by Ellen Byron (2019), "The Pleasures of Eating Alone."

221 *Family stories are important for bonding and maintaining connections:* Barbara Fiese discusses the value of family storytelling and other rituals in a 2006 book, *Family Routines and Rituals*, and in a 2002 article written with colleagues.

Chapter 9: The Good Life at Work: Investing in Connections

223 *"Judge each day"*: The origins of this quote are disputed. It is often attributed to the nineteenth-century Robert Louis Stevenson, but it more likely came a bit later from William Arthur Ward. Stevenson's version is often quoted as, "Don't judge each day by the harvest you reap but by the seeds that you plant." See the following for a discussion of the origin of this quote: https://quoteinvestigator.com/2021/06/23/seeds/#note-439819-1.

228 *On average, workers in the United Kingdom do not work the most hours . . . (belongs to Germany):* Charlie Giattino and colleagues (2013), "Working Hours."

228 *By the time the average individual in the U.K. reaches 80 years of age . . . (13 years!) at work:* Time-use surveys have been completed in many countries. In the U.S. the Bureau of Labor Statistics regularly measures the amount of time people spend on various activities as part of their *American Time Use Survey (ATUS).* These time-use surveys are often used as raw data for calculating estimates of total time spent in activities across the lifespan. These estimates vary depending on the exact data used and the method employed for projections. The illustration we used comes from a post by Gemma Curtis in 2017 (and last modified in April 2021).

228 *63 percent of all Americans age 16 and over are part of the paid labor force:* U.S. Bureau of Labor Statistics (retrieved October 2021), https://data.bls.gov/time series/LNS11300000.

232 *He conducted a study to try to quantify the effects of a difficult workday:* This study is summarized in Schulz and colleagues (2004), "Coming Home Upset: Gender, Marital Satisfaction and the Daily Spillover of Workday Experience into Marriage."

233 *trying to ignore the emotions or hide them . . . often increases their intensity and our body's arousal:* James Gross and colleagues have conducted important research studying the impact on the body of hiding emotions from others. See, for example, Gross and Levenson (1993) and Gross (2002). The research indicates that when individuals actively try to hide emotion from others their cardiovascular system shows signs of arousal and they sweat more (another sign of internal physiological arousal). There is other research (e.g., Hayes and colleagues, 2004) indicating that repeated attempts to ignore or avoid strong negative emotions often result in increases in those emotions and related difficulties.

234 *It's inevitable that we will have hard days at work:* Some people, because of their social or economic status, may have a greater vulnerability to the spillover of negative effects from work to well-being. A 2020 study by Rung and colleagues in Louisiana, for example, suggests that Black women may be particularly vulnerable to spillover of work into family life.

234 *The North End was a heavily Italian neighborhood:* For a history of the Italian immigrant experience in Boston, see Stephen Puleo (2007), *The Boston Italians.*

236 *loneliness increases our risk of death as much as smoking or obesity:* See conclusions in meta-analytic review by Julianne Holt-Lunstad and colleagues in 2010.

236 *Gallup has conducted workplace engagement polls . . . Do you have a best friend at work?:* Annamarie Mann (2018), "Why We Need Best Friends at Work."

236 *people who have a best friend at work are more engaged:* See findings reported by Annamarie Mann (2018) for Gallup and a 1995 study by Christine Riordan

and Rodger Griffeth examining links between friendship opportunities and job satisfaction and engagement.

237 *Positive relationships at work lead to lower stress levels . . . make us happier:* See Mann (2018), article by Adam Grant (2015) in *The New York Times*, and Riordan and Griffeth's 1995 study.

237 *Mary Ainsworth . . . had her own encounters with sexism in the workplace:* Mary Ainsworth wrote about these and other life experiences in a chapter in Agnes N. O'Connell and Nancy Felipe Russo, eds. (1983), *Models of Achievement: Reflections of Eminent Women in Psychology.*

238 *women's roles in the workforce have changed . . . roles in the home:* These trends are documented in Arlie Hochschild's (1989/2012) book, *The Second Shift.* See also the 2000 review by Scott Coltrane documenting similar trends and inequities.

238 *time burdens in the home still weigh more heavily on the woman:* See, for example, work by Bianchi and colleagues in 2012.

244 *On the northeast outskirts of Philadelphia . . . is a large plot of land . . . now being converted into a UPS sorting center:* Inga Saffron (2021), "Our Desire for Quick Delivery Is Bringing More Warehouses to Our Neighborhoods." Additional documentation of these changes can be found at these sites: https://www.inquirer .com/philly/blogs/inq-phillydeals/ne-phila-ex-budd-site-sold-for-18m-to-cdc -for-warehouses-20180308.html; https://www.workshopoftheworld.com/north east/budd.html; and https://philadelphianeighborhoods.com/2019/10/16/north east-residents-look-to-city-for-answers-about-budd-site-development/.

246 *work is a major source of socializing and connection:* See Adam Grant (2015), "Friends at Work? Not So Much."

246 *We became isolated from our workmates, customers, and colleagues:* See 2020 report by Philip Armour and colleagues for the RAND Corporation.

246 *More technological development is inevitable:* For more on the changing nature of certain kinds of work and its implications, see "The IWG Global Workspace Survey" (2019).

Chapter 10: All Friends Have Benefits

250 *"My friends are my 'estate'":* Emily Dickinson wrote this is an 1858 letter to Samuel Bowles.

250 *Ananda, one of the Buddha's disciples:* This quote is from the Upaddha Sutta in the Samyutta Nikaya XLV.2, a translation of which can be accessed here: http:// www.buddhismtoday.com/english/texts/samyutta/sn45-2.html.

250 *"Without friends":* Aristotle wrote this at the beginning of an essay about friendships in the *Nicomachean Ethics* (Book VIII) in 350 BCE.

252 *Seneca wrote . . . "follow into exile":* This quote by Seneca can be found in his *Letters from a Stoic.*

255 *2010 review . . . 148 studies . . . the effect that social connections have on health and longevity:* See 2010 article by Holt-Lunstad and colleagues in *PLOS Medicine* (previously discussed in chapter 2).

255 *A large longitudinal study in Australia . . . strongest network of friends:* See 2004 article by L.C. Giles and colleagues, "Effects of Social Networks on 10 Year Survival in Very Old Australians: The Australian Longitudinal Study of Aging."

256 *study of 2,835 nurses with breast cancer . . . no close friends:* See 2006 article by Candyce Kroenke and colleagues, "Social Networks, Social Support, and Survival After Breast Cancer Diagnosis."

256 *A longitudinal study of over 17,000 . . . decreased the risk of dying:* These results are reported in a 1987 article by Kristina Orth-Gomer and J.V. Johnson, "Social Network Interaction and Mortality. A Six Year Follow-up Study of a Random Sample of the Swedish Population."

258 *"Secret sharing or talking intimately . . . sharing secrets":* This quote comes from a 2013 article (p. 202) by Niobe Way, "Boys' Friendships During Adolescence: Intimacy, Desire, and Loss."

260 *gender differences . . . are smaller than one might expect given our cultural assumptions:* See, for example, Jeffrey Hall's 2011 review and meta-analysis of gender differences in expectations for friendships across thirty-six separate samples with a total of 8,825 individuals. This meta-analysis found that gender differences in expectations for friendships across studies are typically of small magnitude, which means that men and women overlap significantly more in their expectations than they diverge. For example, female participants, on average, expected slightly more out of their friendships than male participants, but the difference was small enough that the distributions for men and women overlap more than 85 percent.

262 *In one fascinating study . . . having a friendly moment with a stranger was uplifting:* These findings come from a 2014 study by Gillian M. Sandstrom and Elizabeth U. Dunn, "Is Efficiency Overrated?: Minimal Social Interactions Lead to Belonging and Positive Affect."

263 *repeated casual contact has been shown to foster the formation of closer friendships:* Jeffrey Hall (2019), "How Many Hours Does It Take to Make a Friend?" presents research on how repeated contact is connected to friendship.

263 *Mark Granovetter has done important research:* Granovetter's classic article on weak ties is "The Strength of Weak Ties" (1973).

267 *"Listening is a magnetic and strange thing":* Brenda Ueland, "Tell Me More."

Conclusion: It's Never Too Late to Be Happy

276 *The typical longitudinal study has a much higher dropout rate . . . entire lifetimes:* In a 2012 study, Kristin Gustavson and colleagues discuss attrition in longitudinal studies.

279 *Courses in social and emotional learning (SEL) . . . are being tested in schools all over the world:* Rebecca Taylor and colleagues review Socio-Emotional Learning interventions in a 2017 meta-analysis. Hoffman and colleagues discuss a leading example of SEL interventions in a 2020 article.

279 *Efforts to bring these same lessons to adults in organizations, workplaces, and community centers are also under way:* We (Bob and Marc) are involved in efforts to promote this kind of learning with adults through our involvement with the Lifespan Research Foundation (https://www.lifespanresearch.org/). Building on the research cited in this book we have created two 5-session courses designed to help individuals lead happier and more satisfying lives. The "Road Maps for Life Transitions" course (https://www.lifespanresearch.org/course -for-individuals/) is designed for adults at all stages of life, while the "Next Chapter" course (https://www.lifespanresearch.org/next-chapter/) is especially designed for individuals between ages 50 and 70.

BIBLIOGRAPHY

Ainsworth, Mary D. "Reflections by Mary D. Ainsworth." In *Models of Achievement: Reflections of Eminent Women in Psychology*, Agnes N. O'Connell and Nancy Felipe Russo, eds. New York: Columbia University Press, 1983.

Aknin, L., et al. "Mental Health During the First Year of the COVID-19 Pandemic: A Review and Recommendations for Moving Forward." *Perspectives on Psychological Science* (January 2022). https://doi.org/10.1177/17456916211029964.

Allen, Joseph P., et al. "Longitudinal Assessment of Autonomy and Relatedness in Adolescent-Family Interactions as Predictors of Adolescent Ego Development and Self-Esteem." *Child Development* 65, no. 1 (1994): 179–94. https://doi.org/10.2307/1131374.

Allibone, Samuel Austin. "Prose Quotations from Socrates to Macauley." Philadelphia: J. B Lippincott, 1880.

Arendt, Hannah. *The Human Condition*, 2nd ed. Chicago: University of Chicago Press, 1958/1998.

Aristotle. *Nicomachean Ethics* 1.5, W. D. Ross, trans. Kitchener, Ontario: Batoche Books, 1999.

Armour, Philip, et al. "The COVID-19 Pandemic and the Changing Nature of Work: Lose Your Job, Show Up to Work, or Telecommute?" RAND Corporation, Santa Monica, CA (2020). https://www.rand.org/pubs/research_reports/RRA308-4.html.

Arrett, Jeffrey J. "Emerging Adulthood: A Theory of Development from the Late Teens Through the Twenties." *American Psychologist* 55 (2000): 469–80.

Bailey, Marlon M. *Butch Queens Up in Pumps*. Ann Arbor: University of Michigan Press, 2013.

Baldwin, T. W. *William Shakespeare's Small Latine and Lesse Greeke*. Urbana: University of Illinois Press, 1944.

Baltes, Paul B. "On the Incomplete Architecture of Human Ontogeny." *American Psychologist* 52 (1997): 366–80.

Bancroft, Anne. *The Wisdom of the Buddha: Heart Teachings in His Own Words.* Boulder, CO: Shambala, 2017.

Bandura, Albert. "The Psychology of Chance Encounters and Life Paths." *American Psychologist* 37, no. 7 (1982): 747–55. https://doi.org/10.1037/0003-066X.37.7.747.

Barreto, Manuela, et al. "Loneliness Around the World: Age, Gender, and Cultural Differences in Loneliness." *Personality and Individual Differences* 169 (2020): 110066. doi:10.1016/j.paid.2020.110066.

Barrick, Elyssa M., Alixandra Barasch, and Diana Tamir. "The Unexpected Social Consequences of Diverting Attention to Our Phones." *PsyArXiv* (October 18, 2020). doi:10.31234/osf.io/7mjax.

Bianchi, Suzanne M., et al. "Who Did, Does or Will Do It, and How Much Does It Matter?" *Social Forces* 91, no. 1 (September 2012): 55–63. https://doi.org/10.1093/sf/sos120.

Birkjaer, Michael, and Micah Kaats. "Does Social Media Really Pose a Threat to Young People's Well-being?" Nordic Council of Ministers (2019). http://dx.doi.org/10.6027/Nord2019-030.

Bohlmeijer, Ernst Thomas, Peter M. ten Klooster, and Martine Fledderus. "Psychometric Properties of the Five-Facet Mindfulness Questionnaire in Depressed Adults and Development of a Short Form." *Assessment* 18, no. 3 (2011): 308–20. https://doi.org/10.1177/1073191111408231.

Bonanno, G. A., et al. "The Importance of Being Flexible: The Ability to Both Enhance and Suppress Emotional Expression Predicts Long-Term Adjustment." *Psychological Science* 15 (2004): 482–87. http://dx.doi.org/10.1111/j.0956-7976.

Bonanno, George, and Charles L. Burton. "Regulatory Flexibility: An Individual Differences Perspective on Coping and Emotion Regulation." *Perspectives on Psychological Science* 8, no. 6 (2013): 591–612. https://doi.org/10.1177/1745691613504116.

Bosma, Hans, et al., "Low Job Control and Risk of Coronary Heart Disease in Whitehall II (Prospective Cohort) Study." *BMJ* 314 (1997): 558–65.

Bromfield, Richard. *Playing for Real.* Boston: Basil Books, 1992.

Buchholz, Laura. "Exploring the Promise of Mindfulness as Medicine." *JAMA* 314, no. 13 (October 2015): 1327–29. doi:10.1001/jama.2015.7023. PMID 26441167.

Buschman, Timothy J., et al. "Neural Substrates of Cognitive Capacity Limitations." *PNAS* 108, no. 27 (July 2011): 11252–55. https://doi.org/10.1073/pnas.1104666108.

Byron, Ellen. "The Pleasures of Eating Alone." *Wall Street Journal*, October 2, 2019. https://www.wsj.com/articles/eating-alone-loses-its-stigma-11570024507.

Cacioppo, John T., Stephanie Cacioppo, and Dorret I. Boomsma. "Evolutionary Mechanisms for Loneliness." *Cognition and Emotion* 28, no. 1 (2014): 3–21. doi:10.1080/02699931.2013.837379.

Cacioppo, John, and William Patrick. *Loneliness: Human Nature and the Need for Social Connection*. New York: Norton, 2008.

Cacioppo, John T., and Stephanie Cacioppo. "The Phenotype of Loneliness." *European Journal of Developmental Psychology* 9, no. 4 (2012): 446–52. doi:10.1080/17405629.2012.690510.

Cacioppo, John T., et al. "The Chicago Health, Aging and Social Relations Study." In *The Science of Subjective Well-Being*, Michael Eid and Randy J. Larsen, eds. New York: Guilford Press, 2008. Chapter 13, 195–219.

Cacioppo, John T., and Stephanie Cacioppo. "The Population-Based Longitudinal Chicago Health, Aging, and Social Relations Study (CHASRS): Study Description and Predictors of Attrition in Older Adults." *Archives of Scientific Psychology* 6, no. 1 (2018): 21–31.

Carnegie, Dale. *How to Win Friends and Influence People*. New York: Simon & Schuster, 1981.

Carroll, Lewis. *Through the Looking-Glass, and What Alice Found There*. London: Macmillan and Co., 1872.

Carstensen, Laura L. "The Influence of a Sense of Time on Human Development." *Science* 312, no. 5782 (2006): 1913–15. doi:10.1126/science.1127488.

Carstensen, Laura L., D. M. Isaacowitz, and S. T. Charles. "Taking Time Seriously: A Theory of Socioemotional Selectivity." *American Psychologist* 54, no. 3 (1999): 165–81. doi:10.1037//0003-066x.54.3.165.

Caspi, A., and T. E. Moffitt. "The Continuity of Maladaptive Behavior: From Description to Understanding in the Study of Antisocial Behavior." In Wiley series on personality processes. *Developmental Psychopathology* 2, *Risk, Disorder, and Adaptation*, D. Cicchetti and D. J. Cohen, eds. Hoboken, N.J.: John Wiley & Sons, 1995.

Chakkarath, Pradeep. "Indian Thoughts on Psychological Human Development." In *Psychology and Psychoanalysis in India*, G. Misra, ed. New Delhi: Munshiram Manoharlal Publishers, 2013, pp. 167–90.

Chamie, Joseph. "The End of Marriage in America?" *The Hill*, August 10, 2021. https://thehill.com/opinion/finance/567107-the-end-of-marriage-in-america.

Coan, James, Hillary S. Schaefer, and Richard J. Davidson. "Lending a Hand: Social Regulation of the Neural Response to Threat." *Psychological Science* 17, no. 12 (2006): 1032–39. doi:10.1111/j.1467-9280.2006.01832.x.

Coan, James. "Why We Hold Hands: Dr. James Coan at TEDxCharlottesville 2013." TEDx Talks, January 25, 2014. https://www.youtube.com/watch?v=1UMHUPPQ96c.

Cohen, Leonard. *The Future*. Sony Music Entertainment, 1992.

Cohen, Shiri, et al. "Eye of the Beholder: The Individual and Dyadic Contributions of Empathic Accuracy and Perceived Empathic Effort to Relationship Satisfaction." *Journal of Family Psychology* 26, no. 2 (2012): 236–45. doi:10.1037/a0027488.

Cohn, Deborah A., et al. "Working Models of Childhood Attachment and Couple Relationships." *Journal of Family Issues* 13, no. 4 (1992): 432–49.

Coltrane, Scott. "Research on Household Labor: Modeling and Measuring the Social Embeddedness of Routine Family Work." *Journal of Marriage and Family* 62, no. 4 (2000): 1208–33. http://www.jstor.org/stable/1566732.

Cox, Rachel Dunaway. *Youth into Maturity*. New York: Mental Health Materials Center, 1970.

Crick, N. R., and K. A. Dodge. "A Review and Reformulation of Social-Information Processing Mechanisms in Children's Development." *Psychological Bulletin* 115 (1994): 74–101.

Cronin, Christopher J., and William N. Evans. "Excess Mortality from COVID and Non-COVID Causes in Minority Populations." *Proceedings of the National Academy of Sciences* 118, no. 39 (September 2021): e2101386118. doi:10.1073/pnas.2101386118.

Curtis, Gemma. "Your Life in Numbers." Creative Commons License, September 29, 2017 (last modified April 28, 2021). https://www.dreams.co.uk/sleep-matters-club/your-life-in-numbers-infographic/.

Czeisler, Mark É., et al. "Mental Health, Substance Use, and Suicidal Ideation During the COVID-19 Pandemic." *Morbidity and Mortality Weekly Report*, United States, June 24–30, 2020: 1049–57. http://dx.doi.org/10.15585/mmwr.mm6932a1.

Dalai Lama. "Economics, Happiness, and the Search for a Better Life." *Dalailama.com*, February 2014. https://www.dalailama.com/news/2014/economics-happiness-and-the-search-for-a-better-life.

Dickinson, Emily. "Dickinson letter to Samuel Bowles (Letter 193)." *Letters from Dickinson to Bowles Archive* (1858). http://archive.emilydickinson.org/correspondence/bowles/1193.html.

Donne, John. *Devotions Upon Emergent Occasions: Together with Death's Duel*. Ann Arbor: University of Michigan Press, 1959.

Dworkin, Jordan. D., et al. "Capturing Naturally Occurring Emotional Suppression as It Unfolds in Couple Interactions." *Emotion* 19, no. 7 (2019): 1224–35. https://doi.org/10.1037/emo0000524.

Eid, Michael, and Randy J. Larsen, eds. *The Science of Subjective Well-Being*. New York: Guilford Press, 2008.

Emerson, Ralph Waldo. "Gifts" (1844). In *Essays and English Traits*. The Harvard Classics, 1909–14. https://www.bartleby.com/5/113.html.

Emerson, Ralph Waldo. *Essays*. Boston: James Munroe & Co., 1841.

Emerson, Ralph Waldo. *Letters and Social Aims*. London: Chatto & Windus, 1876.

Epley, Nicholas, and Juliana Schroeder. "Mistakenly Seeking Solitude." *Journal of Experimental Psychology* 143, no. 5 (2014): 1980–99. doi:10.1037/a0037323.

Erikson, Erik, and Joan M. Erikson. *The Life Cycle Completed: Extended Version*. New York: Norton, 1997.

Erikson, Erik. *Childhood and Society*. New York: Norton, 1950.

Erikson, Erik. *Identity and the Life Cycle*. New York: International Universities Press, 1959.

Fallows, James. "Linda Stone on Maintaining Focus in a Maddeningly Distractive World." *The Atlantic*, May 23, 2013. https://www.theatlantic.com/national/archive/2013/05/linda-stone-on-maintaining-focus-in-a-maddeningly-distractive-world/276201/.

Farson, Richard, and Ralph Keyes. *Whoever Makes the Most Mistakes*. New York: Free Press, 2002.

Fiese, Barbara H. *Family Routines and Rituals*. New Haven: Yale University Press, 2006.

Fiese, Barbara H., et al. "A Review of 50 Years of Research on Naturally Occurring Family Routines and Rituals: Cause for Celebration?" *Journal of Family Psychology* 16, no. 4 (2002): 381–90. https://doi.org/10.1037/0893-3200.16.4.381.

Finkel, Eli J. *The All-or-Nothing Marriage: How the Best Marriages Work*. New York: Dutton, 2017.

Fishel, Anne K. "Harnessing the Power of Family Dinners to Create Change in Family Therapy." *Australian and New Zealand Journal of Family Therapy* 37 (2016): 514–27. doi:10.1002/anzf.1185.

Fraiberg, Selma, et al. "Ghosts in the Nursery: A Psychoanalytic Approach to the Problems of Impaired Infant-Mother Relationships." *Journal of American Academy of Child Psychiatry* 14, no. 3 (1975): 387–421.

Fung, Helene H., and Laura L. Carstensen. "Sending Memorable Messages to the Old: Age Differences in Preferences and Memory for Advertisements." *Journal of Personality and Social Psychology* 85, no. 1 (2003): 163–78.

Gable, Shelly L. "Approach and Avoidance Social Motives and Goals." *Journal of Personality* 74 (2006): 175–222.

Giattino, Charlie, Esteban Ortiz-Ospina, and Max Roser. "Working Hours." *ourworld indata.org*, 2013/2020. https://ourworldindata.org/working-hours.

Giles, L. C., et al. "Effects of Social Networks on 10 Year Survival in Very Old Australians: The Australian Longitudinal Study of Aging." *Journal of Epidemiology and Community Health* 59 (2004): 547–79.

Granovetter, Mark S. "The Strength of Weak Ties." *American Journal of Sociology* 78, no. 6 (1973): 1360–80.

Grant, Adam. "Friends at Work? Not So Much." *New York Times*, September 4, 2015. https://www.nytimes.com/2015/09/06/opinion/sunday/adam-grant-friends-at-work-not-so-much.html?_r=2&mtrref=undefined&gwh=52A0804F85EE4EF9D01AD22AAC839063&gwt=pay&assetType=opinion.

Griffin, Sarah C., et al. "Loneliness and Sleep: A Systematic Review and Meta-analysis." *Health Psychology Open* 7, no. 1 (2020): 1–11. doi:10.1177/2055102920913235.

Gross, James J. "Emotion Regulation: Affective, Cognitive, and Social Consequences." *Psychophysiology* 39, no. 3 (2002): 281–91. doi:10.1017/s0048577201393198.

Gross, James. J., and Robert W. Levenson. "Emotional Suppression: Physiology, Self-report, and Expressive Behavior." *Journal of Personality and Social Psychology* 64, no. 6 (1993): 970–86. https://doi.org/10.1037/0022-3514.64.6.970.

Gustavson, Kristin, et al. "Attrition and Generalizability in Longitudinal Studies: Findings from a 15-Year Population-Based Study and a Monte Carlo Simulation Study." *BMC Public Health* 12, article no. 918. doi:10.1186/1471-2458-12-918.

Hall, Jeffrey A. "How Many Hours Does It Take to Make a Friend?" *Journal of Social and Personal Relationships* 36, no. 4 (April 2019): 1278–96. https://doi.org/10.1177/0265407518761225.

Hall, Jeffrey A. "Sex Differences in Friendship Expectations: A Meta-Analysis." *Journal of Social and Personal Relationships* 28, no. 6 (September 2011): 723–47. https://doi.org/10.1177/0265407510386192.

Hammond, Claudia. "Who Feels Lonely? The Results of the World's Largest Loneliness Study." BBC Radio 4, May 2018. https://www.bbc.co.uk/programmes/articles/2yzhfv4DvqVp5nZyxBD8G23/who-feels-lonely-the-results-of-the-world-s-largest-loneliness-study.

Hanh, Thich Nhat. *The Miracle of Mindfulness: An Introduction to the Practice of Meditation.* Boston: Beacon Press, 2016.

Harris, Judith Rich. *The Nurture Assumption: Why Children Turn Out the Way They Do.* New York: Free Press, 1998.

Hawkley, Louise C., and John T. Cacioppo. "Loneliness Matters: A Theoretical and Empirical Review of Consequences and Mechanisms." *Annals of Behavioral Medicine: A Publication of the Society of Behavioral Medicine* 40, no. 2 (2010): 218–27. doi:10.1007/s12160-010-9210-8.

Hayes, Steven. C., et al. "Measuring Experiential Avoidance: A Preliminary Test of a Working Model." *The Psychological Record* 54, no. 4 (2004): 553–78. https://doi.org/10.1007/BF03395492.

Healy, Kieran. "Income and Happiness." *Kieran Healy* (blog). January 26, 2021. https://kieranhealy.org/blog/archives/2021/01/26/income-and-happiness/.

Helson, R., et al. "The Growing Evidence for Personality Change in Adulthood: Findings from Research with Inventories." *Journal of Research in Personality* 36 (2002): 287–306.

Hill-Soderlund, Ashley L., et al. "Parasympathetic and Sympathetic Responses to the Strange Situation in Infants and Mothers from Avoidant and Securely Attached Dyads." *Developmental Psychobiology* 50, no. 4 (2008): 361–76. doi:10.1002/dev.20302.

Hochschild, Arlie Russell, and Anne Machung. *The Second Shift.* New York: Penguin, 1989/2012.

Hoffmann, Jessica D., et al. "Teaching Emotion Regulation in Schools: Translating Research into Practice with the RULER Approach to Social and Emotional Learning." *Emotion* 20, no. 1 (2020), 105–9. https://doi.org/10.1037/emo00 00649.

Holmes, Thomas H., and Richard H. Rahe. "The Social Readjustment Rating Scale." *Journal of Psychosomatic Research* 11, no. 2 (1967), 213–18. https://doi .org/10.1016/0022-3999(67)90010-4.

Holt-Lunstad, Julianne, Timothy B. Smith, and J. Bradley Layton. "Social Relationships and Mortality Risk: A Meta-analytic Review." *PLoS Medicine* 7, no. 7 (2010): e1000316. https://doi.org/10.1371/journal.pmed.1000316.

Holt-Lunstad, Julianne, et al. "Loneliness and Social Isolation as Risk Factors for Mortality: A Meta-Analytic Review." *Perspectives on Psychological Science* 10, no. 2 (2015): 227–37. doi:10.1177/1745691614568352.

House, James S., et al. "Social Relationships and Health." *Science* New Series 241, no. 4865 (July 1988): 540–45.

Howard, Jane. *Families.* New York: Simon & Schuster, 1998.

Huang, Grace Hui-Chen, and Mary Gove. "Confucianism and Chinese Families: Values and Practices in Education." *International Journal of Humanities and Social Science* 2, no. 3 (February 2012): 10–14. http://www.ijhssnet.com/journals /Vol_2_No_3_February_2012/2.pdf.

Hwang, Tzung-Jeng, et al. "Loneliness and Social Isolation During the COVID-19 Pandemic." *International Psychogeriatrics* 32, no. 10 (2020): 1217–20. doi:10.1017 /S1041610220000988.

Impett, E. A., et al. "Moving Toward More Perfect Unions: Daily and Long-term Consequences of Approach and Avoidance Goals in Romantic Relationships." *Journal of Personality and Social Psychology* 99 (2010): 948–63.

IPSOS. "2020 Predictions, Perceptions and Expectations" (March 2020).

IWG. "The IWG Global Workspace Survey." International Workplace Group (March 2019). https://assets.regus.com/pdfs/iwg-workplace-survey/iwg-workplace-survey -2019.pdf.

Jaffe, Sara. "Queer Time: The Alternative to 'Adulting.'" *JStor Daily*, January 10, 2018. https://daily.jstor.org/queer-time-the-alternative-to-adulting/.

Jeffrey, Karen, et al. "The Cost of Loneliness to UK Employers." New Economics Foundation, February 2017. https://neweconomics.org/uploads/files/NEF_COST-OF -LONELINESS_DIGITAL-Final.pdf.

Jeste, Dilip V., Ellen E. Lee, and Stephanie Cacioppo. "Battling the Modern Behavioral Epidemic of Loneliness: Suggestions for Research and Interventions." *JAMA Psychiatry* 77, no. 6 (2020): 553–54. doi:10.1001/jamapsychiatry.2020.0027.

Jha, Amishi, et al. "Deploying Mindfulness to Gain Cognitive Advantage: Considerations for Military Effectiveness and Well-being." *NATO Science and Technology Conference Proceedings* (2019): 1–14. http://www.amishi.com/lab/wp-content/uploads/Jhaetal_2019_HFM_302_DeployingMindfulness.pdf.

Johnson, Sue. *Love Sense: The Revolutionary New Science of Romantic Relationships.* New York: Little, Brown, 2013.

Kahneman, Daniel, and Amos Tversky. "Prospect Theory: An Analysis of Decision Under Risk." *Econometrica* 47 (1979): 263–91.

Kahneman, Daniel, and Angus Deaton. "High Income Improves Evaluation of Life but Not Emotional Well-being." *Proceedings of the National Academy of Sciences* 107, no. 38 (September 2010): 16489–93. doi:10.1073/pnas.1011492107.

Kiecolt-Glaser, Janice K. "WEXMED Live: Jan Kiecolt Glaser." October 6, 2016, Ohio State Wexner Medical Center. Video, 14:52. https://www.youtube.com/watch?v=hjUW2YC1OYM.

Kiecolt-Glaser, Janice K., et al. "Slowing of Wound Healing by Psychological Stress." *Lancet* 346, no. 8984 (November 1995): 1194–96. doi:10.1016/s0140-6736(95)92899-5.

Killgore, William D. S., et al. "Loneliness: A Signature Mental Health Concern in the Era of COVID-19." *Psychiatry Research* 290 (2020): 113117. doi:10.1016/j.psychres.2020.113117.

Killingsworth, Matthew. "Experienced Well-Being Rises with Income, Even Above $75,000 Per Year." *Proceedings of the National Academy of Sciences of the United States of America* 118, no. 4 (2021): e2016976118. doi:10.1073/pnas.2016976118.

Killingsworth, Matthew, and Daniel T. Gilbert. "A Wandering Mind Is an Unhappy Mind." *Science* 330, no. 6006 (2010): 932. doi:10.1126/science.1192439.

Krause, Sabrina, et al. "Effects of the Adult Attachment Projective Picture System on Oxytocin and Cortisol Blood Levels in Mothers." *Frontiers in Human Neuroscience* 8, no. 10 (2016): 627. doi:10.3389/fnhum.2016.00627.

Kroenke, Candyce H., et al. "Social Networks, Social Support, and Survival After Breast Cancer Diagnosis." *Journal of Clinical Oncology* 24, no. 7 (2006): 1105–11. doi:10.1200/JCO.2005.04.2846.

Kross, Ethan, Ozlem Ayduk, and W. Mischel. "When Asking 'Why' Does Not Hurt. Distinguishing Rumination from Reflective Processing of Negative Emotions." *Psychological Science* 16, no. 9 (2005): 709–15. doi:10.1111/j.1467-9280.2005.01600.x.

Kross, Ethan, et al. (2013). "Facebook Use Predicts Declines in Subjective Well-being in Young Adults." *PLoS ONE* 8, no. 8: e69841.

Kross, Ethan, and Ozlem Ayduk. "Self-Distancing: Theory, Research, and Current Directions." *Advances in Experimental Social Psychology* 55 (2017): 81–136. https://doi.org/10.1016/bs.aesp.2016.10.002.

Kross, Ethan. *Chatter.* New York: Crown, 2021.

Kumashiro, M., and X. B. Arriaga. "Attachment Security Enhancement Model: Bolstering Attachment Security Through Close Relationships." In *Interpersonal Relationships and the Self-Concept*, B. Mattingly, K. McIntyre, and G. Lewandowski Jr., eds. (2020). https://doi.org/10.1007/978-3-030-43747-3_5.

La Fontaine, Jean de. *The Complete Fables of Jean de La Fontaine*. Norman R. Shapiro, ed. Urbana: University of Illinois Press, 2007.

Lazarus, Richard S., and Susan Folkman. *Stress, Appraisal, and Coping*. New York: Springer, 1984.

Lazarus, Richard S. *Emotion and Adaptation*. New York: Oxford University Press, 1991.

Lee, Ellen, et al. "High Prevalence and Adverse Health Effects of Loneliness in Community-Dwelling Adults Across the Lifespan: Role of Wisdom as a Protective Factor." *International Psychogeriatrics* 31, no. 10 (2019): 1447–62. doi:10.1017/S1041610218002120.

L'Engle, Madeleine. *Walking on Water: Reflections on Faith and Art*. New York: Convergent, 1980.

Levesque, Amanda. "The West End Through Time." *Mit.edu* (Spring 2010). http://web.mit.edu/aml2010/www/throughtime.html.

Levinson, Daniel. *The Seasons of a Woman's Life*. New York: Random House, 1996.

Luo, Ye, and Linda J. Waite. "Loneliness and Mortality Among Older Adults in China." *The Journals of Gerontology: Series B* 69, no. 4 (July 2014): 633–45. https://doi.org/10.1093/geronb/gbu007.

Lyubomirsky, Sonja, Kennon M. Sheldon, and David Schkade. "Pursuing Happiness: The Architecture of Sustainable Change." *Review of General Psychology* 9, no. 2 (2005): 111–31. doi:10.1037/1089-2680.9.2.111.

Magan, Christopher. "Isolated During the Pandemic Seniors Are Dying of Loneliness and Their Families Are Demanding Help," *Twin Cities Pioneer Press*, June 19, 2020. https://www.twincities.com/2020/06/19/isolated-during-the-pandemic-seniors-are-dying-of-loneliness-and-their-families-are-demanding-help/.

Mann, Annamarie. "Why We Need Best Friends at Work." Gallup, January 2018. https://www.gallup.com/workplace/236213/why-need-best-friends-work.aspx.

Manner, Jane. "Avoiding eSolation in Online Education." In *Proceedings of SITE 2003—Society for Information Technology and Teacher Education International Conference*, C. Crawford, et al., eds. Albuquerque: Association for the Advancement of Computing in Education (AACE) (2003): 408–10.

Marmot, Michael G., et al. "Contribution of Job Control and Other Risk Factors to Social Variations in Coronary Heart Disease Incidence." *Lancet* 350 (1997): 235–39.

Matthews, Timothy, et al. "Lonely Young Adults in Modern Britain: Findings from an Epidemiological Cohort Study." *Psychological Medicine* 49, no. 2 (January 2019): 268–77. doi:10.1017/S0033291718000788. Epub April 24, 2018.

McAdams, Kimberly, Richard E. Lucas, and M. Brent Donnellan. "The Role of Domain Satisfaction in Explaining the Paradoxical Association Between Life Satisfaction and Age." *Social Indicators Research* 109 (2012): 295–303. https://doi.org/10.1007/s11205-011-9903-9.

McGraw, A. P., et al. "Comparing Gains and Losses." *Psychological Science* 21 (2010): 1438–45.

Moors, A., et al. "Appraisal Theories of Emotion: State of the Art and Future Development." *Emotion Review* 5, no. 2 (2013): 119–24. doi:10.1177/1754073912468165.

Murayama, Kou. "The Science of Motivation." *Psychological Science Agenda*, June 2018. https://www.apa.org/science/about/psa/2018/06/motivation.

Neugarten, Bernie. "Adaptation and the Life Cycle." *The Counseling Psychologist* 6, no. 1 (1976): 16–20. doi:10.1177/001100007600600104.

Nevarez, Michael, Hannah M. Lee, and Robert J. Waldinger. "Friendship in War: Camaraderie and Posttraumatic Stress Disorder Prevention." *Journal of Traumatic Stress* 30, no. 5 (2017): 512–20.

Nielsen Report. "Q1 2018 Total Audience Report." 2018. https://www.nielsen.com/us/en/insights/report/2018/q1-2018-total-audience-report/.

Novick, Tessa K., et al. "Health-Related Social Needs and Kidney Risk Factor Control in an Urban Population." *Kidney Medicine* 3, no. 4 (2021): 680–82.

Oberst, Ursula, et al. "Negative Consequences from Heavy Social Networking in Adolescents: The Mediating Role of Fear of Missing Out." *Journal of Adolescence* 55 (2015): 51–60. https://doi.org/10.1016/j.adolescence.2016.12.008.

Okumura, S. *Realizing Genjokoan: The Key to Dogen's Shobogenzo.* Boston: Wisdom Publications, 2010.

Olsson, Craig A., et al. "A 32-Year Longitudinal Study of Child and Adolescent Pathways to Well-being in Adulthood." *Journal of Happiness Studies* 14, no. 3 (2013): 1069–83. doi:10.1007/s10902-012-9369-8.

Orben, A. "The Sisyphean Cycle of Technology Panics." *Perspectives on Psychological Science* 15, no. 5 (2020): 1143–57. https://doi.org/10.1177/1745691620919372.

Orth-Gomér, Kristina, and J. V. Johnson. "Social Network Interaction and Mortality. A Six Year Follow-up Study of a Random Sample of the Swedish Population." *Journal of Chronic Diseases* 40, no. 10 (1987): 949–57. doi:10.1016/0021-9681(87)90145-7.

Overall, Nickola C., and Jeffry A. Simpson. "Attachment and Dyadic Regulation Processes." *Current Opinion in Psychology* 1 (2015): 61–66. https://doi.org/10.1016/j.copsyc.2014.11.008.

Overstreet, R. Larry. "The Greek Concept of the 'Seven Stages of Life' and Its New Testament Significance." *Bulletin for Biblical Research* 19, no. 4 (2009): 537–63. http://www.jstor.org/stable/26423695.

Park, Soyoung Q., et al. "A Neural Link Between Generosity and Happiness." *Nature Communications* 8, no. 15964 (2017). https://doi.org/10.1038/ncomms15964.

Parker, Kim, et al. "Marriage and Cohabitation in the U.S." Pew Research Center (November 2019).

Pearson, Helen. *The Life Project*. Berkeley: Soft Skull Press, 2016.

Petrova, Kate, and Marc S. Schulz. "Emotional Experiences in Digitally Mediated and In-Person Interactions: An Experience-Sampling Study." *Cognition and Emotion* (2022): https://doi.org/10.1080/02699931.2022.2043244.

Petrova, Kate, et al. "Self-Distancing and Avoidance Mediate the Links Between Trait Mindfulness and Responses to Emotional Challenges." *Mindfulness* 12, no. 4 (2021): 947–58. https://doi.org/10.1007/s12671-020-01559-4.

Plato. *The Symposium*, Christopher Gill, trans. London: Penguin, 1999.

Pressman, S. D., et al. "Loneliness, Social Network Size, and Immune Response to Influenza Vaccination in College Freshmen." *Health Psychology* 24, no. 3 (2005): 297–306. doi:10.1037/0278-6133.24.3.297.

Puleo, Stephen. *The Boston Italians: A Story of Pride, Perseverance and Paesani, from the Years of the Great Immigration to the Present Day*. Boston: Beacon Press, 2007.

Rheault, Magali. "In U.S., 3 in 10 Working Adults Are Strapped for Time." Gallup, July 20, 2011. https://news.gallup.com/poll/148583/working-adults-strapped-time.aspx.

Riordan, Christine M., and Rodger W. Griffeth. "The Opportunity for Friendship in the Workplace: An Underexplored Construct." *Journal of Business Psychology* 10 (1995): 141–54. https://doi.org/10.1007/BF02249575.

Roberts, Max, Eric N. Reither, and Sojoung Lim. "Contributors to the Black-White Life Expectancy Gap in Washington, D.C." *Scientific Reports* 10, article no. 13416 (2020). https://doi.org/10.1038/s41598-020-70046-6.

Roder, Eva, et al. "Maternal Separation and Contact to a Stranger More than Reunion Affect the Autonomic Nervous System in the Mother-Child Dyad: ANS Measurements During Strange Situation Procedure in Mother-Child Dyad." *International Journal of Psychophysiology* 147 (2020): 26–34. https://doi.org/10.1016/j.ijpsycho.2019.08.015.

Rogers, Carl. *On Becoming a Person*. Boston: Houghton Mifflin, 1961.

Rogers, Kenny. "You Can't Make Old Friends." Track 1 on Kenny Rogers, *You Can't Make Old Friends*. Warner Music Nashville, 2013.

Ruavieja. "Ruavieja Commercial 2018 (English subs): #WeHaveToSeeMoreOfEachOther." November 20, 2018. https://www.youtube.com/watch?v=kma1bPDR-rE.

Rung, Ariane L., et al. "Work-Family Spillover and Depression: Are There Racial Differences Among Employed Women?" *SSM—Population Health* 13 (2020): 100724. https://doi.org/10.1016/j.ssmph.2020.100724.

Saffron, Inga. "Our Desire for Quick Delivery Is Bringing More Warehouses to Our Neighborhoods." *Philadelphia Inquirer*, April 21, 2021. https://www.inquirer.com/real-estate/inga-saffron/philadelphia-amazon-ups-distribution

-fulfillment-land-use-bustleton-residential-neighborhood-dhl-office-industrial -parks-20210421.html.

Sandstrom, Gillian M., and Elizabeth W. Dunn. "Is Efficiency Overrated?: Minimal Social Interactions Lead to Belonging and Positive Affect." *Social Psychological and Personality Science* 5, no. 4 (May 2014): 437–42. https://doi.org /10.1177/1948550613502990.

Sandstrom, Gillian M., and Erica J. Boothby. "Why Do People Avoid Talking to Strangers? A Mini Meta-analysis of Predicted Fears and Actual Experiences Talking to a Stranger." *Self and Identity* 20, no. 1 (2021): 47–71. doi:10.1080/15298868 .2020.1816568.

Schulz, Marc, and Richard S. Lazarus. "Emotion Regulation During Adolescence: A Cognitive-Mediational Conceptualization." In *Adolescence and Beyond: Family Processes and Development*, P. K. Kerig, M. S. Schulz, and S. T. Hauser, eds. London: Oxford University Press, 2012.

Schulz, M. S., et al. "Coming Home Upset: Gender, Marital Satisfaction and the Daily Spillover of Workday Experience into Marriage." *Journal of Family Psychology* 18 (2004): 250–63.

Schulz, Marc S., P. A. Cowan, and C. P. Cowan. "Promoting Healthy Beginnings: A Randomized Controlled Trial of a Preventive Intervention to Preserve Marital Quality During the Transition to Parenthood." *Journal of Clinical and Consulting Psychology* 74 (2006): 20–31.

Seneca. *Letters from a Stoic*, trans. Robin Campbell (New York: Penguin, 1969/2004), pp. 49–50.

Sennett, Richard, and Jonathan Cobb. *The Hidden Injuries of Class*. New York: Knopf, 1972.

Shankar, Aparna, et al. "Social Isolation and Loneliness: Relationships with Cognitive Function During 4 Years of Follow-up in the English Longitudinal Study of Ageing." *Psychosomatic Medicine* 75, no. 2 (February 2013): 161–70. doi:10.1097 /PSY.0b013e31827f09cd.

Sharif, M. A., C. Mogilner, and H. E. Hershfield. "Having Too Little or Too Much Time Is Linked to Lower Subjective Well-being." *Journal of Personality and Social Psychology.* Advance online publication (2021). https://doi.org/10.1037/pspp 0000391.

Sheehy, Gail. *New Passages: Mapping Your Life Across Time.* New York: Ballantine, 1995.

Smith, C. A. "Dimensions of Appraisal and Physiological Response in Emotion." *Journal of Personality and Social Psychology* 56, no. 3 (1989): 339–53. https://doi org/10.1037/0022-3514.56.3.339.

Someshwar, Amala. "War, What Is It Good for? Examining Marital Satisfaction and Stability Following World War II." Undergraduate thesis, Bryn Mawr College, 2018.

Spangler, Gottfried, and Michael Schieche. "Emotional and Adrenocortical Responses of Infants to the Strange Situation: The Differential Function of Emotional Expression." *International Journal of Behavioral Development* 22, no. 4 (1998): 681–706. doi:10.1080/016502598384126.

Steinbeck, John. *Travels with Charley: In Search of America.* New York: Penguin, 1997.

Suzuki, Shunryu. *Zen Mind, Beginners Mind: Informal Talks on Zen Meditation and Practice.* Boulder, CO: Shambala Publications, 2011.

Tan, Pia. "The Taming of the Bull. Mind-Training and the Formation of Buddhist Traditions." http://dharmafarer.org/wordpress/wp-content/uploads/2009/12/8.2 -Taming-of-the-Bull-piya.pdf, 2004.

Tarrant, John. *The Light Inside the Dark: Zen, Soul, and the Spiritual Life.* New York: HarperCollins, 1998.

Taylor, Rebecca D., et al. "Promoting Positive Youth Development Through School-Based Social and Emotional Learning Interventions: A Meta-Analysis of Follow-up Effects." *Child Development* 88, no. 4 (July/August 2017): 1156–71. https://doi .org/10.1111/cdev.12864.

Thompson, Derek. "The Myth That Americans Are Busier Than Ever." *theatlantic .com*, May 21, 2014. https://www.theatlantic.com/business/archive/2014/05/the -myth-that-americans-are-busier-than-ever/371350/.

Thoreau, Henry David. *The Writings of Henry David Thoreau (Journal 1, 1837–1846).* Edited by Bradford Torrey. Boston: Houghton Mifflin, 1906.

Twenge, Jean M., et al. "Generational Differences in Young Adults' Life Goals, Concern for Others, and Civic Orientation, 1966–2009." *Journal of Personality and Social Psychology* 102, no. 5 (May 2012): 1045–62. doi:10.1037/a0027408.

Ueland, Brenda. "Tell Me More." *Ladies' Home Journal*, November 1941.

U.S. Bureau of Labor Statistics (retrieved October 2021). https://data.bls.gov/time series/LNS11300000.

U.S. Department of Health and Human Services, Centers for Disease Control and Prevention, National Center for Chronic Disease Prevention and Health Promotion, Office on Smoking and Health. "The Health Consequences of Smoking—50 Years of Progress: A Report of the Surgeon General." Atlanta, 2014. https://www.cdc.gov/tobacco/data_statistics/sgr/50th-anniversary/index.htm.

Vaillant, George. *Aging Well.* Boston: Little, Brown, 2002.

Vaillant, George. *Triumphs of Experience.* Cambridge: Harvard University Press, 2015.

Vaillant, George, and K. Mukamal. "Successful Aging." *American Journal of Psychiatry* 158 (2001): 839–47.

Verduyn, Philippe, et al. "Passive Facebook Usage Undermines Affective Well-being: Experimental and Longitudinal Evidence." *Journal of Experimental Psychology: General* 144, no. 2 (2015): 480–88. https://doi.org/10.1037 /xge0000057.

Verduyn, Philippe, et al. "Do Social Network Sites Enhance or Undermine Subjective Well-being? A Critical Review." *Social Issues and Policy Review* 11, no. 1 (2017): 274–302.

Vespa, Jonathan. "The Changing Economics and Demographics of Young Adulthood, 1975–2016." United States Census Bureau, April 2017. https://www.census .gov/content/dam/Census/library/publications/2017/demo/p20-579.pdf.

Vlahovic, Tatiana A., Sam Roberts, and Robin Dunbar. "Effects of Duration and Laughter on Subjective Happiness Within Different Modes of Communication." *Journal of Computer-Mediated Communication* 17, no. 4 (July 2012): 436–50. https://doi.org/10.1111/j.1083-6101.2012.01584.x.

Waldinger, Robert J., and Marc S. Schulz. "Facing the Music or Burying Our Heads in the Sand?: Adaptive Emotion Regulation in Midlife and Late Life." *Research in Human Development* 7, no. 4 (2010): 292–306. doi:10.1080/15427609.2010.526527.

Waldinger, Robert J., and Marc S. Schulz. "The Long Reach of Nurturing Family Environments: Links with Midlife Emotion-Regulatory Styles and Late-Life Security in Intimate Relationships." *Psychological Science* 27, no. 11 (2016): 1443–50.

Waldinger, Robert J., and Marc S. Schulz. "What's Love Got to Do with It? Social Functioning, Perceived Health, and Daily Happiness in Married Octogenarians." *Psychology and Aging* 25, no. 2 (June 2010): 422–31. doi:10.1037/a0019087.

Waldinger, Robert J., et al. "Reading Others' Emotions: The Role of Intuitive Judgments in Predicting Marital Satisfaction, Quality and Stability." *Journal of Family Psychology* 18 (2004): 58–71.

Wallace, David Foster. "David Foster Wallace on Life and Work." *Wall Street Journal*, September 19, 2008. https://www.wsj.com/articles/SB122178211966454607.

Wang, Wendy. "More Than One-Third of Prime-Age Americans Have Never Married." *Institute for Family Studies Research Brief*, September 2020. https://ifstudies .org/ifs-admin/resources/final2-ifs-single-americansbrief2020.pdf.

Way, Niobe. "Boys' Friendships During Adolescence: Intimacy, Desire, and Loss." *Journal of Research on Adolescence* 23, no. 2 (2013): 201–13. doi:10.1111/jora.12047.

Weil, Simóne. *Gravity and Grace*. New York: Routledge, 2002.

Werner, Emmy, and Ruth. S. Smith. *Overcoming the Odds: High Risk Children from Birth to Adulthood*. Ithaca: Cornell University Press, 1992.

Werner, Emmy E., and Ruth S. Smith. *Journeys from Childhood to Midlife: Risk, Resilience, and Recovery*. Ithaca: Cornell University Press, 2001.

Werner, Emmy E., and Ruth S. Smith. "An Epidemiologic Perspective on Some Antecedents and Consequences of Childhood Mental Health Problems and Learning Disabilities (A Report from the Kauai Longitudinal Study)." *Journal of American Academy of Child Psychiatry* 18, no. 2 (1979): 293.

Werner, Emmy. "Risk, Resilience, and Recovery: Perspectives from the Kauai

Longitudinal Study." *Development and Psychopathology* 5, no. 4 (Fall 1993): 503–15. https://doi.org/10.1017/S095457940000612X.

Whillans, Ashley V., et al. "Buying Time Promotes Happiness." *PNAS* 114, no. 32 (2017): 8523–27. https://doi.org/10.1073/pnas.1706541114.

Whillans, Ashley. "Time Poor and Unhappy." *Harvard Business Review*, 2019. https://awhillans.com/uploads/1/2/3/5/123580974/whillans_03.19.19.pdf.

White, Judith B., et al. "Frequent Social Comparisons and Destructive Emotions and Behaviors: The Dark Side of Social Comparisons." *Journal of Adult Development* 13 (2006): 36–44.

Whitton, Sarah W., et al. "Prospective Associations from Family-of-Origin Interactions to Adult Marital Interactions and Relationship Adjustment." *Journal of Family Psychology* 22 (2008): 274–86. https://doi.org/10.1037/0893-3200.22.2.274.

Wile, Daniel. *After the Honeymoon: How Conflict Can Improve Your Relationship.* Hoboken, NJ: Wiley & Sons, 1988.

Williams, J. M., et al. *The Mindful Way Through Depression.* New York: Guilford Press, 2007.

Wilson, Timothy, and Daniel T. Gilbert. "Affective Forecasting." In *Advances in Experimental Social Psychology.* Mark P. Zanna, ed., vol. 35, pp. 345–411. San Diego: Academic Press, 2003.

Wilson, Timothy D., and Daniel T. Gilbert. "Affective Forecasting: Knowing What to Want." *Current Directions in Psychological Science* 14, no. 3 (June 2005): 131–34.

Wohn, Donghee Y., and Robert LaRose. "Effects of Loneliness and Differential Usage of Facebook on College Adjustment of First-Year Students." *Computers & Education* 76 (2014): 158–67. https://doi.org/10.1016/j.compedu.2014.03.018.

Wolf, Anthony. *Get Out of My Life, but First Could You Drive Me and Cheryl to the Mall?* New York: Farrar, Straus & Giroux, 2002.

Zagorski, Nick. "Profile of Elizabeth F. Loftus." *Proceedings of the National Academy of Sciences* 102, no. 39 (September 2005): 13721–23. doi:10.1073/pnas.0506223102.

Zanesco, Anthony P., et al. "Mindfulness Training as Cognitive Training in High-Demand Cohorts: An Initial Study in Elite Military Servicemembers." *Progress in Brain Research* 244 (2019): 323–54. https://doi.org/10.1016/bs.pbr.2018.10.001.

INDEX

Page numbers in *italics* refer to graphs. Page numbers beginning with 291 refer to notes.